Treating Chronic Pain

The Healing Partnership

Treating Chronic Pain
The Healing Partnership

Aleene M. Friedman, Ph.D.

With a Foreword by
Maurice S. Friedman, Ph.D.

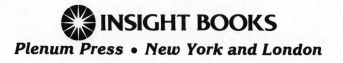

INSIGHT BOOKS
Plenum Press • New York and London

Library of Congress Cataloging-in-Publication Data

Friedman, Aleene M.
    Treating chronic pain : the healing partnership / Aleene M.
 Friedman ; with a foreword by Maurice S. Friedman.
        p.   cm.
    Includes bibliographical references and index.
    ISBN 0-306-44121-7
    1. Intractable pain--Treatment.   I. Title.
    [DNLM: 1. Chronic Disease. 2. Pain--psychology. 3. Pain-
 -therapy. 4. Professional-Patient Relations. 5. Psychotherapy.
 WL 704 F911t]
 RB127.F75   1992
 616'.0472--dc20   ·
 DNLM/DLC
 for Library of Congress   92-3218
                                                                  CIP

ISBN 0-306-44121-7

© 1992 Plenum Press, New York
A Division of Plenum Publishing Corporation
233 Spring Street, New York, N.Y. 10013

An Insight Book

Printed in the United States of America

For Maurice Friedman

My life companion whose writings first inspired me long before we met. We have shared a healing partnership which has been of great importance in my life.

Foreword

Aleene Friedman is a gifted therapist who has brought her understanding of biofeedback and of pain and stress into what has truly been a healing partnership with more than a thousand patients over the last decade. *Treating Chronic Pain* is the product of this experience and of the decades of thinking and research that have made her a pioneer in the new field of "healing through meeting" and in discovering its implications for pain and stress therapy. As a result, she has gone far beyond the behaviorist theoretical model that most people take for granted as associated with biofeedback therapy. Her book represents a breakthrough because in it for the first time chronic-pain therapy and the growing movement of dialogical therapy are integrated into one.

My own expertise entitles me to speak about the second aspect of this breakthrough and not the first. *Healing through Meeting* is the title of a book by the Swiss psychiatrist Hans Trüb and of the introductory essay that Martin Buber wrote for that book when it was posthumously published in 1952. Although all helping relationships and certainly all therapy involve meeting between persons, we can speak properly of healing through meeting only when the relationship between the therapist and the one being helped is central and not ancillary to the healing that takes place. If the psychoanalyst is seen as an indispensable midwife in bringing up material from the unconscious to the conscious, this is not yet healing through meeting. Only when it is recognized that everything that takes place within therapy—free association, dreams, silence, pain, anguish—takes place as a reflection of the vital relationship between therapist and patient do we have what may be properly called healing through meeting.

One of the most important issues that the approach of healing through meeting addresses is the extent to which healing proceeds from a specific healer and the extent to which healing takes place in the "between"—in the relationships between therapist and client, among the members of a group or family, or even within a community. When it is the last of these, is there a special role, nonetheless, for the therapist as facilitator, midwife, enabler, or partner in a "dialogue of touchstones"? Another issue is the extent to which we are talking about a two-sided event that is not susceptible to techniques in the sense of willing and manipulating in order to bring about a certain result.

Another important problem that healing through meeting encounters is that of the limits of responsibility of the helper. Therapists open to the new vistas of healing through meeting will feel that more is demanded of them than their professional methods and their professional role provide. What is crucial is not the skill of the therapist but, rather, what takes place between the therapist and the client and between the client and other people. This has important implications for our understanding of the subtitle of this book: *The Healing Partnership*. Only as a partner can a person be perceived as an existing wholeness. To become aware of a person, as Martin Buber has pointed out, means to perceive his or her wholeness as a person defined by spirit: to perceive the dynamic center that stamps on all utterances, actions, and attitudes the recognizable sign of uniqueness. Such an awareness is impossible if, and as long as, the other is for me the detached object of my observation, for that person will not thus yield his or her wholeness and its center. It is possible only when he or she becomes present for me in genuine dialogue.

Although in my writings I have dealt with quite a range of thinkers who have contributed to our understanding of "healing through meeting," the only books written to date that stand at the center of the developing movement of dialogical therapy are Hans Trüb's *Healing through Meeting* (1952), Leslie H. Farber's *The Ways of the Will: Toward a Psychology and Psychopathology of the Will* (1966), my own books *The Healing Dialogue in Psychotherapy* (1985) and *Dialogue and the Human Image: Beyond Humanistic Psychology* (1991), and Richard Hycner's *Between Person and Person: Toward a Dialogical Psychotherapy* (1991). Aleene Friedman's *Treating Chronic Pain: The Healing Partnership* may now be added to that small but growing list.

One of the theoretical bases of Aleene Friedman's integration of pain therapy and healing through meeting is her recognition that, more than any other experience, pain involves us in the unmaking and making of the world, as Elaine Scarry states in her book *The Body in Pain*. Aleene Friedman has gone decisively beyond Scarry, however, in following Martin Buber's understanding of "the world" as that common cosmos that we build together through our common "logos"—that common speech-with-meaning to which we contribute, each from our own unique place, in a strenuous "tug of war." Recognizing this, Aleene Friedman understands not only how pain can isolate one from the common world but also how it is the healing partnership alone that can bring the chronic pain sufferer back into the common world.

This insight is one that Aleene Friedman spells out explicitly only in her last chapter. In the preceding chapters she lays the groundwork of our understanding of the healing partnership, of the "dialogue of touchstones" (my own phrase), and of chronic pain, and she does so with rich, in-depth case studies from her own experience as a therapist and that of others. Although it is not usually considered fitting for one who stands in close personal relationship to someone else to make such a judgment, I believe the result is an extraordinary book that will have great appeal to professionals of many fields and to laypersons everywhere. For which of us do not have to live with chronic pain during some periods of our lives, and which of us do not long for that healing partnership that may not "cure" the pain but may enable us to bring ourselves into meaningful relationship with it and, in so doing, lessen its isolating and intolerable aspects?

Maurice S. Friedman

Preface

Beginnings and endings eventually flow into one another over the years, but the healing partnerships that have come into being in the past are very much a part of the present. I am indebted to all those who have been with me from the beginning and to those who have journeyed with me along the way, especially my three sons, Ron, Chris, and Ken Dorn, who have given me unconditional love.

It has been over twenty-five years since I first met Professor Camille Brown at UCLA. She provided me with a healing partnership that has enhanced both my personal and academic life. Whatever I have accomplished over the years is very much related to her teachings and personal integrity.

The theoretical foundations on which this book rests are the thoughts of Martin Buber and Maurice Friedman. Their writings have had a great impact both on my present work as a pain therapist and during my years as a teacher in the Los Angeles School District.

I am grateful to my friend Laurel Mannen for preparing the manuscript for this book. I also wish to express my gratitude to all my patients in the healing partnership over the years with whom I have discovered the insights that enabled me to write this book.

Contents

CHAPTER 1

Old Wounds—New Healing

The emphasis in this book is on healing, not as a technique to be learned, but as a way of being in partnership. The healing partnership begins with the conviction that the human spirit cannot be reduced to a predictable variable, to be determined and controlled to achieve a particular outcome. The complexities of our state of health are intricately bound with the multiplicity of our life stories, and these complexities cannot be examined as separate entities. We are, as human beings, subject to an interdependency that is, from the beginning of our lives, the very fabric of our existence.

Scientists search for answers and provide us with clues. The promise of science is that there are answers that will simplify the complexities that initiate and sustain the state of our health. Yet healing arises from within, and occurs most often in response to the meetings with others in daily life. Healing is a dynamic phenomenon that defies absolute predictability; it is a mystery that never fully reveals itself. It is an integral part of living, a possibility for all human beings throughout their lifetimes.

We all sustain wounds to our beings, and these wounds affect the quality of our lives. We do not exist in terms of a separate body and a mind, but rather as an integration of both. What affects one part of our being has an impact on the whole. To be wounded is to suffer an assault upon our sense of self—upon our whole being. These assaults may result in temporary or permanent changes in the way we conduct our lives. Wounds build up layer by layer throughout our lifetime. Some may heal while others lie dormant, but unhealed. Accidents, other traumas, and the failure of relationships all serve to add new wounds and to awaken old ones. One may reach the limits of one's resources, and as a result the delicate balance between wellness and disease—life and death— may be adversely affected.

To heal is to restore wholeness, yet life is in a constant flux, and there is no former wholeness that can be regained. Each wounding causes a new configuration, and each period of healing is a time of gaining renewed resources and a new wholeness that arises out of the present.

The most obvious wounds are those resulting from physical traumas that produce visible injuries, or symptoms that arise from detectable physical abnormalities. These wounds indicate the presence of a disease entity or a life-threatening disorder. Here there is an organic component, which many see as being limited to the physical. Yet woundedness, as I use the term, goes beyond the division of mind and body, encompassing all of the assaults upon our selfhood—our human spirit. Loneliness, grief, failed relationships, isolation, and loss inflict wounds that are every bit as serious as the disease entities that they may precipitate. Wounding affects us physically and emotionally, and one aspect of our being cannot be separated from the other. Too often, healing is equated with the elimination of obvious symptoms, while the less obvious wounds remain untreated and unhealed.

Symptoms or other outward signs of a disease, injury, or trauma may no longer exist, but the effects of the wounding may take months, years, or a lifetime to heal. It is also possible that a person may be healed without the elimination of all symptoms. One may even experience this healing during the moments before death. I was witness to a dying woman's last meeting with her family. She was with her son and his wife, her grandson and his wife, and her newly born great-grandson. The ravages of cancer had left her very weak, but she was able to cradle her great-grandson for a short time. She looked peaceful, and with her eyes she bade farewell to each family member. She was not cured of her symptoms, but I do feel that whatever wounds she may have borne over the years were, at that moment, healed. That evening this woman, whom I had met during the last weeks of her life, died a peaceful death. I will never forget the beauty of those last moments with her and her family.

I never did meet the 10-month-old boy who was reported cured by a staff psychologist. The infant had, for no apparent reason, developed an eating disorder that involved gagging and/or regurgitating when he ate. The psychologist had the child hospitalized, and a mild electric shock was administered every time he gagged or regurgitated. Ten days later, the boy was pronounced cured and sent home. He had been cured of his symptoms, and the psychologist was obviously proud of his success, but I question whether this child's experience was a healing one. His treatment, and the lack of follow-up care, may have left him with wounds that will fester during the years to come. These untreated wounds may diminish his capacity to withstand a future trauma.

What I am discussing here is related to stress, and there is a point where accumulated stress, or even a single event, becomes an assault upon our sense of self. Such a trauma might be regarded as a strain on the whole organism, leaving the person wounded and lacking in wholeness. This state of being can be conceived of as a rift in "The Partnership of Existence." It has to do with a disturbance in our sense of self in relation to others. It is my belief that it is here that our deepest wounds are sustained. The potential for healing lies in the development of "healing partnerships" that enhance the sense of wholeness and the ability to bring this wholeness into relationship with others. When this wholeness is lacking, there is likely to be increased pain and suffering.

When they experience persistent discomfort or unusual symptoms, most people seek professional help. The first meeting between the professional and the patient is an important part of the healing process. In my own work, I have often witnessed the nonhealing and sometimes damaging results of treatment that lacks a personal relationship. This is illustrated by the experiences of Margo L., a patient who was referred to the medical clinic where I was working, after two years of unsuccessful treatment in other areas of the country.

Margo's primary complaint was redness, itching, tenderness, and burning sensations in the pelvic area and on the inside of her upper right and left leg areas. These post-surgical symptoms had worsened over the previous year, and other symptoms, unrelated to this problem, had also worsened during this period. These included headaches, neck and shoulder pain, low back pain, and a frequent state of agitation.

Margo made all of the necessary arrangements for a complete evaluation of her symptoms, and was initially referred to an internist. He examined her and referred her to a gynecologist, who referred her to a dermatologist, who referred her to a rheumatologist. Each specialist examined her in the context of his own particular specialty, and in some cases diagnostic tests and/or X rays were ordered. The patient returned to the internist, who informed her that there appeared to be no treatable organic cause for her symptoms. He recommended a psychiatric consultation and a revisit in one month.

After a brief psychiatric consultation, Margo was given a prescription for tranquilizers and a referral to the pain treatment department. There she was required to take a psychological test, and was then seen by a staff psychologist. Margo spoke to the psychologist about her symptoms, and began to express some personal concerns about her present life situation. The psychologist stated that her psychological test results had revealed all that he needed to know about her, and went so far as to imply that her test results revealed more than she herself could reveal to him. Margo's angry response to this statement was deemed inappropriate behavior, and was seen as further evidence of her contributing psychological problems.

Later that day, Margo reported to my office for a session of pain therapy. She was feeling angry and discounted, and this first session was devoted to the effects of these feelings. Only afterwards could we go on to address the problems that had necessitated her initial referral for pain treatment.

Despite a poor prognosis, Margo improved. She learned to slow down her respiration rate, to decrease muscle tension, to use visualization techniques, to begin to develop her own resources for healing, and to realize that she was capable of doing so. She brought to each meeting her courage, sense of humor, self-awareness, and a desire to improve her state of health. Margo was willing to take some of the responsibility for her current health problems, and to engage actively in the development of a program to achieve her goals. I contributed guidance and my professional resources. These resources were the raw material with which we worked, but only with this relationship did we determine which aspects of the treatment program were best suited to Margo's needs. (Refer to Chapter 13 for more on Margo's case.)

The healing partnership does not demand that the patient meet the healing professional's expectations. Margo's improvement was dramatic, but she had days when she seemed to be losing ground. She needed to know that this, too, was a normal part of her progress. She kept in touch after leaving the program and returned after one year for a short "refresher course." Margo was never fully "symptom free," but she no longer feared her symptoms. She was facing many life issues that her physicians had not wanted to hear about. Her aged parent was chronically ill, demanding, and needing more attention. Her husband was being treated for several serious health problems, and there were many problems in their relationship. She had valid concerns about her future, but she continued to work to improve her day-to-day life.

Health care that does not fully address the person being treated is often economically damaging as well as nonhealing. The patient's symptoms may actually be exacerbated by a consultation with someone who does not personally respond to the patient's own unique identity. Every person has the right to expect professional care that is healing, even when there is little hope of eliminating the symptoms. It is within the healing arts that the promise of healing lies, and where it is formally practiced. When a person seeks professional care, it is a demonstration of faith in the healer. This faith is best served when the healer has, in turn, a belief in the patient's own capacity for healing. When this occurs, healing becomes a shared responsibility and a mutual effort.

Listening and being present for the other person is, in itself, a healing act. It is a sharing of one's common humanity, and does not carry with it the expectation of easy solutions to complex life issues. The healing partnership is built on trust and mutual respect. This grows out of the initial meeting between the patient and the professional. The patient needs to be heard, and his or her own truth respected. There are always time constraints, but the time spent with patients needs to be their time. You cannot listen to a patient if you are evaluating everything that he or she is saying, and if you do this, you may miss those issues that are most important to the patient.

One day, at a department meeting, a staff member turned to me and said, "Whatever you did to Margo really worked, but don't tell me what it was." He would not have understood that I did not "do something" to Margo, but rather worked in partnership with her. This particular psychologist's professional treatment model was behavioral psychology, and it was not the patient, but the model that determined his way of meeting each patient. He believed that only the professional knows what is best for the patient. He was, however, perplexed by the fact that approximately fifty percent of patients do not follow professional advice, and many of these patients manage to get well on their own.

Each individual needs to be met where he or she stands in relation to the wholeness of their being. This approach does not represent a further division between medicine, psychology, and the various other non-medical approaches to healing, but is rather a stance that views healing as dialogical. The emphasis is on the "meeting" with the other as a central element of healing: "healing through meeting." Healing is not the sole domain of one professional group. Teachers, social workers, parents, and most other members of society are capable of enhancing healing, and many do just that.

Modern medicine, during this century, has developed increasingly powerful drugs and advanced technological skills. In psychotherapy, the emphasis has been on the development of testing devices and schools that promote a particular type of psychotherapeutic technique. What has been left out is a consideration of the extent to which healing occurs in the "between," in the therapist/patient relationship. This important aspect of the healing process has generally been ignored in favor of an emphasis on scientific advancement. What is needed is a shift in emphasis from technique to dialogue. "The meaning of dialogue is not found in either one or the other of the partners, nor in both added together, but rather in their exchange."[1] The dialogue is of value in itself, and is not merely a way to attain a particular goal.

> The dialogue about how one is can only be couched in human terms, familiar terms, which come easily and naturally to all of us; and it can only be held if there is a direct and human confrontation, an "I–Thou" relation between the discoursing worlds of physicians and patients.[2]

The concept of "healing through meeting" has usually been applied to psychotherapy, but as evidenced in the writings of Oliver Sacks and many other physicians, there is a growing awareness of the need for physicians to go beyond medical technology and to relate to the patient as a unique human being. In the article "Needed: A New Way to Train Doctors," Harvard President Derek Bok stated, "Doctors themselves can influence the course of sickness and cure by their behavior toward patients."[3]

President Bok noted that one-third to one-half of all patients seeking medical advice from their primary care physician have no physical (or biomedical) ailment at all. I have observed that most of these patients are dismissed without being heard. In doing this, the physician is dismissing the fact that grief, social conditions, guilt, lifestyle, and loneliness can all adversely affect health. To minister to the spirit may, in some cases, provide a measure of preventive medicine. President Bok stated that physicians need to " . . . understand the emotional, psychological, and cultural underpinnings of human behavior, including the interweaving of mind and body in illness and health." He also suggested that future physicians be taught "the familiar skills of listening, observing, interviewing, and communicating effectively."[4] "Healing through meeting" unites the person with his or her world, and healing takes place in the "between" of the meeting. The realm of the "between" is not limited to one type of healer, but is the domain of all healers who dare to enter into dialogue with their patients.

Why, with the advanced medical technology and pharmacology and the multitude of psychological strategies that are available, do I choose to emphasize the meeting between person and person as the focal point of healing? One has only to look at our society to see that the need for healing is endemic. Much of our sickness lies in the lack of caring relationships, our isolation from one another, and the losses that leave us wounded and alone in our suffering. Science and technology can never replace the need for a loving touch or a glance that speaks more directly than words. The usefulness of science and technology cannot be negated, but when I meet and affirm a fellow human being in our common humanity, it is a step towards establishing a wholeness within that person that restores the human spirit. This is where healing begins.

> Kinship is healing; we are physicians to each other. . . . The essential thing is feeling at home in the world, knowing in the depths of one's being that one has a real place in the home of the world.[5]

In his book *The Broken Heart: The Medical Consequences of Loneliness*, James J. Lynch documented how the effects of social isolation, the lack of human companionship, death or absence of parents in early childhood, sudden loss of love, and chronic human loneliness are significant contributors to premature death. His focus was on heart disease, but he commented that "almost every cause of death is significantly influenced by human companionship."

> ... we shall concentrate on premature death due to heart disease simply because it is the leading cause of death and as such can be used to help illustrate the fact that health and human companionship do go together. In this regard, coronary heart disease is no different from any other cause of death. Cancer, tuberculosis, suicide, accidents, mental disease—all are significantly influenced by human companionship ... Nature uses many weapons to shorten the lives of lonely people. On a statistical basis it simply chooses heart disease more frequently.[6]

Dr. Lynch advocates the taking of individual medical–social life histories, which may be less "objective," but present a fuller picture of the patient's present state of health and potential for illness.

Wounds and the strain they cause can lead to premature death through disease or a sudden-death syndrome. They may lead to a chronic state of unwellness, including psychological disorders or one of a multitude of chronic pain problems. It is my premise that in order to decrease the effects of these wounds, we must move beyond the bounds of the traditional medical model of treatment. If people are getting well by using yoga, acupuncture, meditation, biofeedback, placebos, humor, dialogue, and imagery, then we need to look at what this means in terms of healing. Bernard Siegel, M.D., an Assistant Clinical Professor at Yale University Medical School, stated:

> Medicine is a failure-oriented specialty, in which we produce mechanics and life-savers ... medicine needs to stop trying to fight death, and instead teach people how to live ... We ought to study the patients who didn't die when they were supposed to: to spend time with them, learn from them. Historically that is what medicine did. The physician was there to share in the patient's life, and the physician and patient participated as a team ...

> When a patient's prognosis is not good, I say to people, "Whom do you love—call them up and say it." "You have conflicts, call and

resolve them." Get everything ready, and then—as one patient said—"I felt so good I didn't want to die." I'd like to teach people that now, not wait until they're almost dead.[7]

Physicians have been trained to expect results from specific medications and medical interventions. What they refer to as "placebos" are the indirect, nonspecific interactions that are not fully understood, but do appear to facilitate healing. Herbert Benson, M.D., stated that numerous studies have shown that belief is an important aspect of the placebo effect.

When we dissected the placebo effect a number of years ago, we found three basic components: one, the belief and expectation of the patient; two, the belief and expectation of the physician; and three, the interaction between the physician and the patient. When these are in concert, the placebo effect is operative.[8]

In his book *Awakenings,* Oliver Sacks beautifully illustrated the need to address the uniqueness of each patient.

Diseases have a character of their own, but they also partake of our character; we have a character of our own, but we also partake of the world's character: character is monadic or microcosmic, worlds within worlds within worlds, worlds which express worlds. The disease–the man–the world go together, and cannot be considered separately as things-in-themselves.[9]

Healing occurs beyond the bounds of traditional medicine, and also incorporates the meeting between person and person. When we meet others and address their uniqueness, their potential for healing is enhanced. When the meeting is between a patient and a helping professional, the primary responsibility for meeting the other is from the professional's side of the relationship; the potential for a healing partnership emanates from that side. This cannot be planned in advance, but arises out of the moment and is, in all cases, a personal response that addresses the uniqueness of the other.

A dialogical relationship between helper and patient demands a different type of approach, involving more than the use of technique, drugs, or medical procedures. Maurice Friedman states:

> Only as a partner can a person be perceived as an existing wholeness. To become aware of a person means to perceive his or her wholeness as persons defined by spirit: to perceive the dynamic center that stamps on all utterances, actions, and attitudes the recognizable sign of uniqueness. Such an awareness is impossible if, and so long as, the other is for me the detached object of my observation; for that person will not thus yield his or her wholeness and its center. It is possible only when he or she becomes present for me.[10]

The healing partnership unites medical technology with an earlier wisdom: The realization that healing is not accomplished by medicine alone, but through the meeting between patient and healer. The consideration of illness is removed from the strict confines of pathogenic disease: loneliness, grief, loss, trauma, anger, anxiety, and many other factors are considered. Each partner in the healing relationship is responsible for bringing his or her own resources to the meeting with the other. There is no guarantee that a healing relationship will emerge, but an opening way is established. This gives rise to the possibility of a healing partnership.

Predictable results would be reassuring, but the human condition offers no such assurances. When we stand in relation to the other and are present in the fullness of our being, the potential for human wholeness in partnership is enhanced, and we know more fully what it means to be human.

Notes

1. Maurice Friedman, *The Confirmation of Otherness in Family, Community and Society* (New York: The Pilgrim Press, 1983), p. 6.
2. Oliver Sacks, *Awakenings* (New York: Harper Perennial, 1990), p. 225.
3. Derek Bok, "Needed: New ways to train doctors," *Harvard Magazine*, (May–June, 1984), pp. 32–43.

4. Ibid., pp. 70–71.
5. Oliver Sacks, *Awakenings* (New York: Harper Perennial, 1990), p. 272.
6. James J. Lynch, *The Broken Heart: The Medical Consequences of Loneliness* (New York: Basic Books, Inc., 1979), p. 4.
7. Bernard Siegel, "The health of the healing profession: An interview with Bernard Siegel," *Revision*, Vol. 7, No. 1 (Spring 1984), pp. 87–93.
8. Herbert Benson, "Looking beyond the relaxation response: An interview with Herbert Benson," *Revision*, Vol. 7, No. 1 (Spring 1984), pp. 50–54.
9. Oliver Sacks, *Awakenings* (New York: Harper Perennial, 1990), p. 229.
10. Maurice Friedman, *The Healing Dialogue in Psychotherapy* (New York: Jason Aronson, 1985), p. 4.

CHAPTER 2

The Healing Partnership

"Healing through meeting" is the greatest gift that one person can give to another. What occurs between the healer and the one to be healed is seldom addressed. It is not a therapeutic technique, but rather the " . . . unfolding of the sphere of the between, or that which Martin Buber refers to as the 'dialogical.'" It is here that partnership of existence takes place, and it is here that healing occurs.

To meet the other as a partner is to be willing to meet the person in his or her uniqueness. This is impossible if I view the other as an object to be studied. Only when I see the "other" is his or her wholeness revealed; when this occurs, it is an act of confirmation. This does not mean that I accept everything about the other, but it does mean that I confirm the other in his or her own uniqueness.

When I meet with patients I listen, and I try to imagine, from their side, what is real for them. This does not mean that I give up my own ground, but that I practice what is known as "inclusion." Maurice Friedman states:

> In contrast to both empathy and identification, inclusion means a bold imaginative swinging "with the intensest stirring of one's being," into the life of the other so that one can, to some extent, concretely imagine what the other person is thinking, willing, and

feeling and so that one adds something of one's own will to what is thus apprehended ... It means ... grasping them in their uniqueness and concreteness.[1]

Inclusion is vital to the development of a dialogical relationship. In the relationship between the healing professional and patient, it is the professional who takes the bold step over to the patient's side of the dialogue. Full maturity between the professional and the patient is impossible, and may place an undue burden on the patient: the patient comes to the professional for help. While there may be some mutual healing, it is not the responsibility of the patient to heal the professional. If the patient is seen by the professional as an object to be "known," "healing through meeting" will not take place. But if the patient does not have the resources to meet the professional in his or her wholeness, "healing through meeting" may still take place.

These healing encounters are not limited to the sphere of the health professional; they are possible in all meetings between people. The focus here is on the health professional's meeting with a patient, because it is in this situation that healing is most often sought. Each person, however, is part of a larger community; the healing that takes place between the patient and the professional must also take place between the patient and the other persons in his or her life. A healing partnership is influenced by the whole of the other's existence.

> The one between cannot totally make up for the place of the other. No amount of therapy can be of decisive help if a person is too enmeshed in a family, community, or culture in which the seedlings of healing are constantly choked off and the attempts to restore personal wholeness are thwarted by destructive elements of the system.[2]

The therapist must accept the patient as he or she is at that moment. But it is also important to move beyond this initial stance of acceptance to one of concern with the patient's becoming the unique person he or she is called to become. Confirmation is not static. The initial confirmation is just the beginning of the development of existential trust and existential healing. The therapist cannot know the potential of the patient. Patterns of illness may have been the patient's only way to cope with a very destructive family and/or social situation. In the beginning, it is important to listen to and acknowledge the patient's point of view. The therapist "imagines the real" during this listening period. But he or she must, in time, help the patient resume a dialogue with the community. This means to " . . . place upon the patient the demand of the community."[3] The patient must move through both of these stages for healing to occur.

I have learned to listen, and my patients have taught me that there is no single source of present pain and suffering. Some patients, when asked how long they have hurt, stated that they have hurt all of their lives. Others identify a specific causal factor; yet there will be other factors which exacerbate symptoms or interfere with the healing process.

Medical charts, patients histories, and psychological tests all provide general information about a patient, but it is the patient's own voice that opens the way. It is an act of confirmation to listen to a patient and act on his or her concerns. In a recent article, John Pfeiffer noted that many patients are lost because the health professional does not take the time to listen to the patient. Physicians and their patients were videotaped during regular office visits, and in 52 of the 74 interviews, the physician was more interested in the time allotted to each patient than in the patients themselves.

> . . . doctors interrupted their patients a mean time of 18 seconds after they had begun describing their problems. Half of the patients were interrupted right after mentioning the first symptom. Later, when some of the doctors who participated in the study listened to themselves, they explained that their interruptions were in the interest of time. But the interviews fail to support this notion. Patients generally reported two to four symptoms and when interrupted, finished within a minute.[4]

Doctors also tended to interrupt after the first symptom was mentioned, because they thought that the first symptom was diagnostically the most important. Yet frequently this is not the case. There are often psychosocial factors which are totally ignored, in deference to the initial physical complaint. It may take time to discover a patient's real concerns, and this time is seldom allotted.

It has been estimated that between 30 and 70 percent of symptoms are overlooked or misdiagnosed.[4] This estimate resulted from studies by Susan Block, a psychiatrist and internist at Harvard Medical School. She stated that doctors tend to overlook or ignore headaches, fatigue, and restlessness "... that stem from psychological causes like anxiety or depression." She noted that more than one prescription may be warranted, and that "empathy, encouragement, and discussion of the options are important to a successful therapeutic program."

Quality health care depends on the willingness of both patient and professional to engage in an honest exchange. The need for education on both sides is vitally important, and symptoms need to be addressed in relation to the unique situation of the individual patient.

> Medical practitioners, by failing to incorporate cultural, financial, job, family, and personal needs into the therapeutic program, are constructing unsuccessful treatment programs ... Americans make some 600 million office visits per year: More than half the cases are "nonsymptomatic" ... Clearly doctors are being called on increasingly to respond to people needing more than medicine.[5]

To begin to grasp the essence of another human being, one must provide time for that person to share his or her own uniqueness. This does not imply that a demand be placed on the patient, but rather that there be an opportunity for the patient to make a personal response that arises from the moment.

Each relationship with a patient is unique. The issues of mutuality and inclusion, the limits of responsibility of the helper, and the development of a healing relationship cannot be planned out in advance. It is within the relationship itself that these issues are addressed, and, as in all meetings, there may be a failure to develop a viable relationship. This is the risk that one takes when one reaches out to meet the other, but this risk-taking awakens the possibility of "real living."

There is no such thing as a typical patient. John M. brought his concerns to our first meeting. He had requested biofeedback and pain-therapy sessions after being discharged from an inpatient treatment program. He had a history of depression, headaches, upper back pain, and anxiety attacks. He was very clear about the fact that he wanted to learn how to decrease or eliminate his daily anxiety attacks. John had been in group therapy, behavior modification classes, and individual psychotherapy. His other symptoms were under control, but the anxiety attacks disrupted his family and social life. During our first meeting we discussed his symptoms, possible warning signs, what was most likely to trigger his symptoms, and what, if anything, had helped him in the past. We needed to develop a working relationship, and to establish a ground of meeting. We developed an agenda, but it was an open agenda that took form over time and was brought into being through our combined efforts.

In John's life, fears had begun to take precedence over strengths. John feared being out of control; and the more he feared his symptoms, the more vulnerable he became. During our time together we explored ways for John to use his internal resources. The very processes that created the anxiety attacks could be reversed to help him prevent and/or reduce his symptoms. In time, he learned to control his breathing to calm himself, to relax his neck, shoulders, and upper back muscles, to focus on a quieting phrase, and to practice these techniques on a daily basis.

John's symptoms improved, but his ability to tolerate time constraints continued as an ongoing issue. Even his young son's natural enthusiasm created a sense of demand that often triggered an anxiety attack. As John began to share some of his personal history, both the sources and the complexities of his condition began to emerge.

John carried with him the scars of childhood trauma. His parents were members of a religious community in Germany, one that believed in the merits of corporal punishment. Both at home and at school, there were demands for perfection and very few rewards for accomplishment. The members of this community did not believe in traditional medical care, and when John was severely injured at the age of eight, they turned to home care and prayer. A physician was called only when it appeared that John was dying, and the physician determined that it was too late to administer medical treatment. John remembered a near-death experience, but it was many years before he could verbalize what he had felt at that time.

After graduating from high school, John left home and worked his way through college. He eventually married and had two children. He only returned to his parent's home once, to visit his dying mother. He kept in touch with his brother, but made no effort to continue contact with his father.

Over the years John became increasingly demanding and critical of his family members, and he physically abused his children. After twelve years of marriage, his wife divorced him and obtained custody of their children. John was alone and he hated what he had become and above all he feared that this was now the core of his being.

John felt that he had failed himself, and he wanted a second chance. In particular, he wanted another child and the opportunity to establish a loving relationship with this child. In time he did remarry, and his son was born a year later. He hoped that this child would help him to break the cycle of family violence, but he did not know how to handle his increased anxiety. This brought us back to his main reason for seeking professional help.

Healing relationships come into being in their own time. They can be facilitated, but they cannot be forced. My relationship with John was based on trust, honesty, and a belief in his ability to reduce his symptoms. As he shared his personal history he was also sharing what Maurice Friedman would call his "touchstones of reality." Our touchstones of reality are developed from the events in our lives, and come into being when we fully respond to that which reaches out to meet us in our wholeness. This is not an objective discourse, but a sharing of what is uniquely our own.

In order to have real contact with one another, we must overcome our "education": for we are programmed to "hear" in such a way that we rarely really hear. Most of our education is an education in the methods of abstracting. Consequently, we do not hear the person who speaks, but only his "opinion" or "point of view."[6]

What is especially important about the "dialogue of touchstones" is that it offers an alternative to the either/or way of thinking. The person is not thought of as being divided into a mind and a body, or as being totally well or totally sick. When John shared his touchstones, he was sharing his own unique reality. It is not easy to share one's touchstones. There is often a fear of revealing what may be considered the inner self as opposed to the outer, or social, self. This fear, and this dichotomy between the inner and the outer self, blocks the dialogue of touchstones. In time, without this dialogue, one's touchstones tend to atrophy. The person is then cut off from himself/herself and from the community.

Such a person needs the help of someone who can glimpse and share the unique reality that has come from this person's life experience and can help this person find a way of bringing it into the common order of existence so that he or she too may raise what he or she has experienced as I into the communal reality of "We." ... Such persons need the help of a therapist who can "imagine the real" and practice inclusion in order to help them enter into a dialogue of touchstones.[7]

The healing relationship comes into being when the otherness of the patient is not only respected, but is enhanced by the therapist. When a patient is trusting enough to reveal a part of himself/herself, it is a gift—one that should not be objectified and categorized as a way to separate the "healthy" therapist from the "sick" patient. Many of the patients whom I see already feel that they are "sick," and have given up hope of ever being well. Yet when there is a dialogue of touchstones, there is usually a healing effect. The initial touchstones may reveal past experiences of pain, but in time there is also an unfolding of the resources that have sustained the patient. More positive touchstones may be revealed or forged from the therapeutic experience itself. When a dialogue of touchstones takes place, each partner touches the other in a way that may or may not involve actual physical touching. Both patient and therapist are affected, and the dichotomy between health and illness becomes less of an issue.

One problematic factor that can interfere with the dialogue of touchstones is the denial of the patient's own touchstones. This is often encouraged by families, therapists, physicians, and others who may feel that their opinion is the only one of any value. We often learn to say what we feel we should say, and thus our uniqueness is lost. We are all impoverished when a voice is silenced because it does not fit into another's world view. Each person, by sharing a part of his or her world, shares a part of his or her humanity, and this touches on our common humanity.

In sharing his touchstones with me, John shared his strengths and his vulnerabilities. He had, over the years, chosen life over death, and he did feel that he had been given a second chance to heal his past. He also began to realize that it was not his young son's responsibility to heal him, but that their relationship was a healing one. John developed calming images and breathing patterns that decreased his symptoms. He became less fearful of his symptoms and more in touch with his own needs.

At his wife's suggestion, John and his family visited his elderly father. Despite the fact that it was an intercontinental trip and the travel arrangements involved both train and flight schedules, John managed quite well. Shortly after arriving at his father's home, John's young son climbed up on his grandfather's lap and kissed his cheek. John's father held his grandson and wept, saying that he had never felt loved, and he had not learned how to express affection. For the first time in his life, John understood his father's suffering and pain. He also realized that he did not need to punish others or himself for the suffering that had been inflicted upon him. He was not miraculously healed, but it was a healing experience.

Time does not heal wounds. Like the scars on John's body, the wounds remain, and they must be acknowledged and somehow incorporated into one's being. This is most likely to happen when there is a genuine meeting that creates a bond between spirits.

The help of the therapist is not, in the first instance, a matter of finding the right words, still less techniques of communication. It is a matter of the dialogue of touchstones coming into being between one who cannot reach out and one who can . . . It might be called "Healing through meeting," or even "a dialogue of touchstones." For that is the secret of the bond between spirit and spirit.[8]

John was not repaired and he was not restored, but there was healing. It was he who decided that he was ready to continue working on his own, but he also knew that he could schedule additional appointments, if necessary. I saw John once after he left the program, and I called him after a period of several months. He was participating in a regular exercise program, and was using what he had learned on a daily basis. John had completed several home projects, and his relationship with his wife, his children from his previous marriage, and his young son were less fraught with anxiety. He visited with his brother on a regular basis, but was unwilling to develop friendships outside his own family circle. He had dreams and hopes for the future, and there was no reason to doubt his capacity to bring these aspirations to fruition.

Medical and psychological tests are often designed to determine deficits. What may be right with the person is generally given very little attention, because the focus is on what is wrong with the person. The person is viewed outside the context of his or her life situation; thus the person's basic humanity is not evident to the examiner. Often no credit is given for how well the patient may be coping, or for his or her own power as a person. If we look at people only in terms of the impersonal statistical data that are collected during a testing period, it is difficult to gain a sense of them as fellow human beings who are attempting to establish a meaningful life despite various deficits and imperfections. Oliver Sacks points out that meaning comes from many sources, and as long as we look for the defects, we may not find that which is intact and functioning. He calls for a science of the concrete—a return to the narrative.

When Oliver Sacks writes about a patient, there is a respect for the patient's integrity; his or her point of view is a vital part of the reporting process. More often, the opposite is true. The patient's voice is silenced or discounted, and the attitude is one of viewing the patient as a defective human organism that must be repaired and somehow restored, if possible, to a healthier state. While this may sound like a very worthwhile endeavor, it is based on a one-sided view of what the professional determines is best for the patient. This approach may account for the fact that over 50 percent of patients seen by physicians do not comply with the medical prescriptions that are given to them.

I know of no one who more perfectly exemplifies the clinical application of "healing through meeting" than Oliver Sacks. He refers to the need to heal the split between psychology and neurology, stating that this split has existed since the turn of the century. Freud, Babinski, and Tourette were, according to Sacks, " . . . the last of their profession with a combined vision of body and soul, 'It' and 'I,' neurology and psychiatry." This split has, according to Sacks, resulted in a soulless neurology and a bodiless psychology. Sacks suggests that a return to the tradition of the clinical narrative is imperative if we are to include the "who" as well as the "what" in the patient case study.[9]

Oliver Sacks introduces the notion that, "perhaps the need to find or feel some ultimate harmony or order is a universal of the mind, whatever its power, and whatever form it takes." Science has been built on one particular concept of order, and it is within this abstract world that many of the answers to our health and social problems are sought. What has been left out is the concrete, the particular, the person himself/herself. Patients are attempting to put harmony and order back into their lives, but the means they use may be very destructive or we may think that they are harmful. I believe that before any judgment is made, one must listen to the patient, not as a scientist, but as a caring professional who is willing to engage in a healing dialogue. In this way, patients are participants in their own healing process, and they share some of the responsibility and the credit for healing.

Dialogue with the patient opens up the realms of healing that reestablish order through art, music, dance, exercise, and the integrity of the patient's own touchstones of reality. To utilize the patient's touchstones of reality is to help him or her to use those resources that are uniquely the patient's own. This, I believe, is the essence of the healing dialogue. Here, the parameters of healing are broadened beyond those of surgery, pharmacology, and schools of therapy and wholeness and health take on a new meaning. Dancing, art, and other forms of movement can provide us with active visualizations and renewed images of ourselves.

Our self concepts are often static and the self-images we form become fixed and block new responses. Only in dialogue are we able to bring our touchstones forth in relationship to the present. What arises from any meeting is the result of what each partner is able to bring to the meeting, each according to his/her own resources; this designates the limits of the partnership.

Notes

1. Maurice Friedman, *The Healing Dialogue in Psychotherapy* (New York: Jason Aronson, 1985), p. 198.
2. Ibid., p. 3.
3. Ibid., p. 139.
4. John Pfeiffer, ed., "Listening for emotions," *Science 86*, Vol. 8, No. 5 (June 1986), p. 14.
5. Ibid., p. 16.
6. Friedman, *Healing Dialogue*, p. 207.
7. Ibid., p. 217.
8. Ibid., pp. 217–218.
9. Oliver Sacks, *The Man Who Mistook His Wife for a Hat and Other Clinical Tales* (New York: Harper and Row, 1987), p. xiv.

CHAPTER 3

Establishing a Healing Dialogue
Clinical Applications

Respecting the integrity of the patient provides the groundwork necessary for the establishment of a healing partnership. The patient's point of view is a vital part of the initial patient/therapist meeting. Oliver Sacks states that we need to include the "who" as well as the "what" in the patient case study.

> To restore the human subject at the center—the suffering, afflicted, fighting, human subject—we must deepen a case history to a narrative or tale: only then do we have . . . a real person, a patient, in relation to disease—in relation to the physical.
> The patient's essential being is very relevant to the higher reaches of neurology, and in psychology; for here the patient's personhood is essentially involved, and the study of disease and of identity cannot be disjoined. Such disorders, and their depiction and study, indeed entail a new discipline, which we may call the "neurology of identity," for it deals with the neural foundations of the self, the age-old problem of mind and brain.[1]

Rebecca

In one of his own narratives, Sacks refers to a young woman named Rebecca. When he first tested Rebecca, he classified her as severely retarded and noted that she had been described by various other people as a "motor moron."

> When I first saw her—clumsy, uncouth, all-of-a-fumble—I saw her merely, or wholly, as a casualty, a broken creature, whose neurological impairments I could pick out and dissect with precision: a multitude of apraxias and agnosias, a mass of sensorimotor impairments and breakdowns, limitations of intellectual schemata and concepts similar (by Piaget's criteria) to those of a child of eight. A poor thing, I said to myself, with perhaps a "splinter skill," a freak gift, of speech; a mere mosaic of higher cortical functions, Piagetian schemata—most impaired.
>
> The next time I saw her, it was all very different. I didn't have her in a test situation, "evaluating" her in a clinic. I wandered outside; it was a lovely spring day, with a few minutes in hand before the clinic started, and I saw Rebecca sitting on a bench, gazing at the April foliage quietly, with obvious delight. Her posture had none of the clumsiness which had so impressed me before. Sitting there, in a light dress, her face calm and slightly smiling, she suddenly brought to mind one of Chekov's young women—Irene, Anya, Sonya, Nina—seen against the backdrop of a Chekovian cherry orchard. She could have been any young woman enjoying a beautiful spring day. This was my human, as opposed to my neurological, vision.[2]

Tests, as Sacks points out, are most often designed to determine deficits. What may be right is generally given very little attention because the focus is on what is wrong with the person. Then, too, as pointed out in the above quotation, the person is viewed outside the context of their life situation, and their basic humanity is not evident to the examiner. The patient is not given credit for how well he or she may have been coping, or for his or her own power as a person. In the case of Rebecca, Sacks relates how it was Rebecca who showed the way toward a program that helped her to develop the many talents that had not been evident during the initial testing period. Rebecca moved beautifully to music and she excelled in drama. She was placed in several workshops and classes that were designed to improve her cognitive skills, but they totally ignored her own creative abilities. Rebecca decided to quit the classes because, in her words, "they do nothing to bring me together." Rebecca loved the theater and she enrolled in a theater group. She became, in Sacks's words, a complete person, and while she was performing it was not evident that she was mentally defective. Rebecca wanted to have meaning in her life, and that meaning was achieved through her performances in the theater. She became a successful actress, and while she was on the stage, it was not evident that she was retarded.

If we look at people only in terms of the impersonal statistical data that is collected during a testing period, it is difficult to gain a sense of them as fellow human beings who are attempting to establish a meaningful life despite various deficits or other imperfections. Sacks pointed out that meaning comes from many sources; as long as we look for the defects, we may not find that which is intact and functioning. He calls for a science of the concrete—a return to the narrative.

When Oliver Sacks writes about his patients, there is a respect for the integrity of the patient, and the patient's point of view is a vital part of the reporting process. More often, the opposite is true.

I have talked with many of my own patients who have sought professional advice, but who failed to comply with the various prescriptions that were given to them. In some cases, they did not want to take medications, or they could not relate to the treatment plan. Some patients found their health professional slow to respond to their post-treatment complaints or questions and simply decided, on their own, what they should do, or they sought further advice. Some patients felt that they had failed to respond as they should have and simply looked for other alternatives or decided to accept their suffering. Many patients may not realize that health professionals often have their own "pet cures." This may be a particular medication, an exercise program, or a particular therapy technique. One neurologist, where I once worked, prescribed Yoga and swimming for almost every patient that he saw. One of the referring psychologists warned every patient that they wouldn't get well if they didn't start jogging or doing aerobics every day. These were health-oriented prescriptions, but they were seldom, if ever, discussed in relation to the individual patient. Other options were not discussed, and the age, general condition of the patient, and their openness to such programs were not addressed. What is even more unlikely to happen is for the health professional to consult the patient in relation to the patient's own needs. Sometimes the patient simply needs the validation that they are actually doing quite well or the assurance that their symptoms are not life threatening. When the uniqueness of the patient is lost during the search for a diagnosis and treatment plan, the patient's humanity is diminished.

Sacks's statement that the narrative element is seldom found in medical reports has been borne out in my own work. Medical reports are usually very sterile and devoid of the personal psychosocial material that elaborates on the humanity of the patient. The following case history illustrates this point, but it would be possible to use most other patient case materials to accomplish this same end.

Ray

Ray was first brought to the clinic when he was 18 months old for evaluation of growth retardation. It is noted in the chart that he had grown normally until he was 4 or 5 months old, but that he was now in the 3rd percentile for height and weight expectations for his age. His 4-year-old sibling was in the 90th percentile for her age and had grown normally since birth. Other relevant data included the type and amount of growth hormones that had been administered before coming to the clinic and the effects of these drugs on Ray's growth. Ray's present height and weight, as well as the height of his mother, father, and grandparents, were also listed. Ray has unusually small ears and this congenital abnormality was mentioned twice. The fact that he has Arnold–Chiari malformation (a hydrocephalic condition that did not require drainage) was not mentioned. Skeletal X rays were deemed to be normal, and the final diagnosis was constitutionally retarded growth. Thyroid medications were prescribed, and the next consultation entry occurred almost sixteen years later.

Ray was 17 years old when he himself consulted a doctor at the clinic about his growth potential. He had grown about 2 inches each year for the past few years and was approximately 5 feet 3 inches tall and weighed 125 pounds. Since being examined as a toddler, he had been in good health except for occasional headaches, and he had suffered a concussion when he was 14 years old. He had developed acne during his teenage years and took daily medication for this condition. The chart notes stated that both parents were in good health, but that his mother suffered from migraine headaches and that his father and sister both had allergies. All physical signs appeared to be normal, and puberty had started when he was about 13 years old.

Ray was 22 years old when he again consulted a physician at the clinic. His symptoms were visual disturbances, muscle weakness on the right side of the face, and occasional headaches. It was noted that he had mild dyslexia and mild-to-moderate ventricular dilation but no other significant abnormalities. At the conclusion of this consultation, the attending physician felt that the possibility of a brain-stem tumor could be ruled out as a source of Ray's symptoms. In the actual report, Ray's name was never mentioned—he was referred to as a 22-year-old man. Six months after his initial examination, Ray's symptoms worsened and a magnetic resonant imaging study revealed a brain-stem/pontine glioma. Radiation therapy was recommended and this was started soon after the diagnostic workup was completed.

As soon as it was determined that Ray had a tumor, his family met and worked out a ten-step program that was aimed at helping Ray to "overcome." This program was sent to Ray's neurologist, and her support was requested. The following steps were listed:

1. Radiation therapy
2. Rest, sleep, and relaxation
3. Top-notch nutrition
4. Vitamin and mineral supplements
5. Visual imagery program
6. Exercises
7. Keeping busy: school and friends
8. Laughter (Norman Cousins's approach)
9. Positive outlook: visualizing success
10. Prayer

The family was very interested in the possibilities of Ray's using visual imagery to help reduce or eliminate his tumor.

Ray's father, John, at one time had been my patient for several months, but he had seldom mentioned his son. He was concerned with learning to handle his job-related stress more effectively and to decrease his frequent "sinus pressure headaches." On the few occasions that he had mentioned Ray, there was some concern about his learning difficulties in relation to his hydrocephalic condition. Ray had always been in regular classroom situations, and a small private college had been selected so that he would have a better chance of succeeding in college.

John was generally a quiet, private person, but as soon as he became aware of Ray's tumor, he made an appointment to see me and we discussed the impact of this news on his family and on himself. We discussed the ten-step program that the family had worked out, and he said that Ray was aware of his condition but wanted to keep his life as normal as possible. He asked me to set up a series of biofeedback sessions for Ray, and this is how I came to meet him.

As Sacks has stated in his writings, medical charts seldom give the reader a sense of the person that is to be treated. I read Ray's chart and I saw pictures of his tumor and one picture of him that had been taken to illustrate the eye/facial involvement that had resulted from the tumor pressing on the optic nerve. When Ray arrived for his first appointment, I saw a boyish young man of short stature but solidly built. He had his hair combed forward and appeared to be covering a receding hairline; his ears were small and his right eye did not appear to be functioning well. During the first session, we discussed Ray's school schedule, his interests, and his goals. We also discussed the purposes of the treatment program and areas of concern. I learned that Ray liked being with his friends and that he planned to keep living on campus. He had told his friends about the tumor, but he was trying to keep his life as normal as possible. He liked sports, his sociology class, and good food. He did not like having the radiation treatments and was tired and nauseous after the treatments.

During the first meeting, it was easiest to see, in Sacks's words, the deficits: mild speech impediment, ear deformity, eye and facial muscle weaknesses, and small stature. By the end of the session, however, the assets began to emerge and Ray's sense of humor, honesty, hopes for the future, and his willingness to tackle each new challenge were evident. We had decided to work on general relaxation, warming techniques, and imagery. I would be seeing Ray once a week after his radiation treatments.

One of Ray's immediate concerns was his discomfort before and during radiation therapy sessions. The sessions were usually short, but he felt anxious before the session, and his position on the table, during the session, was not comfortable. Occasionally, he had to stay in the same position for up to an hour, and he was facing at least four weeks of radiation treatment. The after-effects, as mentioned earlier, were fatigue and nausea, and Ray was afraid that he might not be able to keep up with his class assignments. He had decided to cut down on his class load, but he wanted to remain a student and to stay involved in some of the activities at school. Concerns about his studies interfered, to some degree, with scheduling regular times to practice the biofeedback techniques, but he was very receptive to the treatment program.

One of my first tasks, during the initial treatment session, was to introduce relaxation/breathing techniques. Once Ray was able to utilize these skills, we went on to visual imagery. Ray used his relaxation skills to diminish his feelings of anxiety before the radiation treatments, but he also wanted an effective way to reduce his discomfort during the treatment period. We decided to develop a visual image that he could focus on during his time on the radiation treatment table, and he came up with an image that incorporated, for him, all the elements of a great vacation spot. This image proved to be especially helpful during the longer sessions on this very uncomfortable table, and it appeared to help Ray develop a greater acceptance of the radiation treatment program.

Visual imagery was the most important part of our treatment program. Our next task was to develop an image related to the tumor site itself. We discussed various possibilities, but Ray himself came up with what he felt was best for him. He saw the tumor as a large snowball and he decided that he would melt it away. We had been working on warming techniques and this was another way to use this very effective self-regulation technique. We were still in the process of working with Ray's tumor-reduction image, but it should be remembered that imagery and the development of self-regulation skills were only two aspects of the much larger total health care program, which also included the ten-step program that Ray and his family had developed.

Ray took an active part in his own treatment program, and I feel that his active participation contributed to a high level of compliance. The future was very uncertain for Ray. His tumor was thought to be benign (or possibly cancerous); because of the tumor location, an operation to remove the tumor or a biopsy was impossible. What was certain was the fact that Ray loved life, and he had managed to obtain the most out of his life. He had not focused on his deficits, but neither had he failed to take them into consideration in terms of his future goals and his daily activities.

Several months after my last meeting with Ray, I left the country for an extended stay abroad. When I returned home I did not return to my previous workplace. Contact with my former patients was, for the most part, cut off. I had seen at least a thousand patients over the years. Memories of many of these patients were little more than an indiscriminate blur, but memories of others, such as Ray, remained clear and continued to have an impact upon the direction of my present work.

I waited over a year to call Ray's home to inquire about his health. The last inquiry, before leaving for my trip abroad, had produced a reassuring report. Ray was doing well at school; his tumor appeared to be in remission and he was still incorporating some of the self-regulation/imagery techniques. I had a happy ending to hold onto and I was aware of the fact that I did not want to disturb this status quo. Eventually, I did call Ray's father and he told me that Ray had died about a year earlier. Ironically, he had not died from the effects of his tumor. Rather, he had died from an infection that occurred after a procedure designed to relieve some pressure that had developed from his long-dormant hydrocephalic condition.

In my mind, Ray's death is in no way a failure. It was I who had to be reminded that it is not the "happy ending" that counts, but rather the struggle to make each day a meaningful event. Ray did not demand a healthy state. He dreamed of the future but lived in the moment. Ray brought to the treatment sessions a wholeheartedness that implied a belief in his future. He called me out as a person and our meetings drew on our mutual resources. I was his guide and teacher, but he too contributed to the process. Ray's sensitivity and willingness to confront even a life-threatening situation deeply affected my own life. His parents' love and caring also touched on my own feelings as a parent and in terms of the trust that was inherent in their request for my help. Ray's death made me very sad, but I am gratified that I had an opportunity to work with him and to know him as a person.

The patient deserves to be treated as more than a statistical notation. Weight, height, past illnesses, present complaints, neurological responses, and occupational and/or educational data are only the beginning points, but too often they are the whole basis for determining the "who" and the "what" of the patient. It is possible that the potentials for healing may be revealed through the dialogical, and it is quite evident that the healing process is often diminished by a failure to meet the patient while acknowledging his wholeness and uniqueness.

Science has been built on one particular concept of order, and it is within this abstract world that many of the answers to our health and social problems are sought. What has been left out is the concrete, the particular, the person. Patients are attempting to put harmony and order back into their lives, but the means may, in some cases, be or appear to be very destructive. Before this judgment can be made, it is, I believe, very important to listen to the patient, not as a scientist, but rather as a caring professional who is willing to engage in a healing dialogue. In this way, the patients are participants in their own healing process, and they share some of the responsibility as well as the credit for healing.

I am reminded of a physician whom I once called in to minister to my 80-year-old grandmother. She was feeling ill and I was not sure how serious the symptoms were, so I wanted her to be examined. The physician spent about 20 minutes examining my grandmother, and then he spoke to me about her condition. He stated that there were multiple causes for concern, but that she was basically functioning well despite his findings. He felt that any aggressive medical testing and/or treatment plans would probably cause more problems than she was currently having. "Your grandmother," he stated, "lives in a delicate balance between health and illness, and I do not want to disturb this balance unless it is absolutely necessary." My grandmother lived another ten years and required very little medical attention during that time. Many of my own patients seek reassurances about their health or desire help that is related to their own lifestyle, age group, and emotional resources.

I believe that Sacks shows the way toward a clinical treatment program that widens the parameters of healing beyond surgery, pharmacology, and schools of therapy. Dialogue with the patient opens up the realms of healing that reestablish an order related to the integrity of the patient's own touchstones of reality. To utilize the patient's touchstones of reality is to help him/her to use those resources that are uniquely his/her own. This, I believe, is the essence of the healing dialogue. In the case of Rebecca, Sacks shows how drama was her touchstone of reality and how it helped her to attain a state of wholeness and health.

> What we see, fundamentally, is the power of music to organize— and to do this efficaciously (as well as joyfully!) when abstract or schematic forms of organization fail. Indeed, no other form of organization will work . . . And in drama there is still more—there is the power of role to give organization, to confer, while it lasts, an entire personality. The capacity to perform, to play, to be, seems to be a "given" in human life, in a way which has nothing to do with intellectual differences. One sees this with infants, one sees it with the senile, and one sees it, most poignantly, with the Rebeccas of this world.[3]

Patricia Norris, former president of the Biofeedback Society of America and a clinical psychologist at the Menninger Clinic, adds what I believe to be an additional dimension to the concept of "healing through meeting." She and her former patient, Garrett Porter, wrote *Why Me? Harnessing the Healing Power of the Human Spirit.* This book served as a model for my work with Ray, and it is, for me, another excellent example of the application of the concept of "healing through meeting." Norris based her book on an earlier paper, "The Role of Psychophysiologic Self-Regulation in the Treatment of Cancer: A Narrative Case Report."

Norris believes that both the patient and the professional are participants in the healing process and that both share the responsibility for healing. She notes that many physicians feel that the treatment program is their responsibility and this alleviates the patient's sense of guilt if the treatment program does not succeed in healing the patient. Norris points out that there can be no failure in trying. "Everyone can be a success at trying, and trying brings strength and energy of its own, which is a healing force." Trying brings hope into what may appear to be a hopeless situation, and as we have seen in my work with Ray, in the work of Oliver Sacks, and now in the work of Patricia Norris, it is possible to bring hope into the treatment plan if the goals are not limited to what the medical model might view as success. Sacks's patients were not cured, and some of Norris's patients have died from the effects of their cancer, but in most cases there was a sense of healing and, most important, the establishment of some sense of being a part of life as a whole. To be healthy is not always to be free of disease or a disabling condition, but rather to be living the best life that one can live at any given moment.

> None of us can postpone death forever, and a cure does not confer immortality on anyone, and yet this often seems to be the unconscious agenda of both physician and patient. Perhaps this is at the root of the great fear of conveying false hope to a patient. How could hope ever be false? In this life, there are never any guarantees, and this is especially true for people facing catastrophic and life-threatening illness. But there is always hope for something. Hope for a better day, for more comfort, for some joy and fun. Hope for less pain. Even hope for a more aware, more comfortable death, closure with loved ones accomplished.[4]

We are continually acting on the conscious and unconscious images that we hold in relation to ourselves. The work of Freud, Jung, and Assagioli provided much of the groundwork for a psychophysiological view of healing. Patricia Norris incorporates a dialogical approach in her work with visualization and self-regulation and exemplifies the possibilities for healing when both the patient and the health professional fully participate in a healing relationship. The emphasis is on helping the patient to gain a sense of empowerment and self-mastery, both physiologically and psychologically. For this to take place, both the patient and the health professional must believe that healing is possible. This belief is directly related to the development of visualizations that are aimed at creating images of healing and wellness.

> Our behavior is controlled by the visualizations we hold, consciously or unconsciously. If we wish to change some aspect of our life, we must first become aware of the images we hold and then create visualizations for the changes we wish to see come into being.[5]

The concepts of imagery and self-regulation are well known in what we refer to as primitive cultures and in the Far Eastern cultures. The importance of imagery and the possibilities of self-regulation have, however, been generally ignored in Western medicine.

> Imagery precedes thought phylogenetically and developmentally ... and I believe that imagery initiates all thought processes, associations, and all secondary-process thinking.
>
> Now, in work with visualization and healing, it becomes obvious that imagery precedes physiological action within the body as well as action in the world.[6]

As mentioned earlier, Western medicine has tended to ignore the implications of imagery in relation to health and the possibilities that self-regulation affords the patient both in preventive health care and in the treatment of illness. The issues that have been mentioned are patient responsibility in regard to the treatment program and patient guilt when the treatment program fails to produce a state of wellness. Another issue is the powerful stance that the medical/psychological community assumes when they take the major responsibility for patient care and the results of that care. What is missing here is a shared responsibility for the treatment program between the health professional and the patient. This, I believe, involves a dialogical approach to healing, and the health professional must be willing to meet the other on the other's ground while still maintaining his or her own ground. The patient becomes more than a statistical/diagnostic notation, and it is here that the images and touchstones of the patient are revealed and may, in some cases, be reformed through the confirmation of a caring relationship.

Garrett

In her work with 10-year-old Garrett Porter, Patricia Norris demonstrates how she and Garrett used the principles of self-regulation, imagery, and dialogue to help rid Garrett of his life-threatening brain tumor.

> At that time, Garrett was a "Trekkie," in love with Star Trek, Battlestar Galactica, and the whole idea of space exploration. He organized the scenario for his visualization around the space drama. . . . My role was Ground Control, and by this device, we maintained a constant dialogue on the tape, creating the visualizations as we went along. . . . In addition to this symbolic visualization, Garrett developed an organic, biological visualization. Eventually, he came to use the organic visualization most of the time.[7]

The organic visualization involved Garrett walking, as a tiny being, through his brain. When he approached the tumor, he saw it as disorganized and powerless. He would then see his white cells attacking and destroying his tumor. Garrett was, during this period, under the care of several physicians and supportive staff. He was not showing any improvement despite an excellent treatment program, and he was given a year to live. Despite this prognosis, Garrett continued to use his visualization techniques, and, one day, he was unable to see his tumor during the "brain walk." Garrett was sure that the tumor was gone, but it took some time to verify this fact scientifically.

Norris points out that Garrett's battle with cancer moved back and forth between progress and decline.

> In the taping, Garrett ran all the sound effects. He had set the board up previously with the battleships all concealed. Each time he unleashed an attack against the planetoid, we really did not know whether it would be a hit or a miss. This turned out to be fortuitous. This is how life really is. Every day is not equally good, and every attack is not equally effective. Garrett experienced good days and not so good days, but from the beginning he seemed aware that if he felt bad or did poorly one day, he could improve the next.[8]

It is very easy for a patient to become discouraged when he or she has a period of increased symptoms, and a part of the ongoing dialogue is to establish that the flow of life is not an even, forward movement. Symptoms do not disappear but, rather, tend to recede, and it may be necessary to establish some type of vigilance that gives warning signals when the symptoms are returning to the foreground of our existence.

Visualization, imagery, biofeedback-assisted self-regulation, and deep relaxation were basic to Garrett's treatment program. He has, over the years, continued to maintain some aspects of this program as a preventive measure. Honesty and openness were also important, and it is here that dialogue is facilitated. My own experience bears this out. The more I work with patients, the more I come to realize that healing is accomplished within a healing relationship. Garrett had to make the decision that he wanted to live, but he needed openness and responsiveness in order to explore this issue. Fear, tension, and suppression of feelings tend to increase symptoms. Patients need safe environments that reduce their fears and above all environments that respect their individual humanity. There are times when illness or death are conscious choices, and this too must be respected.

The Healing Dialogue

Dancing, art, and other forms of movement provide us with active visualizations and possibly renewed images of ourselves. It is also evident that the more static visualizations that we create in our mind form images of ourselves. These images relate to our touchstones of reality, and only in dialogue are we able to bring them forth in relation to the present. Both Sacks and Norris have demonstrated the importance of the dialogical relationship in healing. When there is a meeting between the patient and the health professional, there can be no ready-made remedy. What comes forth from any meeting is the result of what each partner is able to bring to the meeting according to his or her own resources, and this determines the limits of the partnership.

The therapeutic value of dance, art, music, exercise, and other forms of dialogue demonstrate the fact that healing goes far beyond pharmacology, surgery, and therapeutic techniques. I do not know the cardiologist who treated an elderly friend some years ago, but I liked his prescription. My friend had suffered a slight stroke and the doctor treated him in the more traditional way. But then he recommended to my friend that he take up square dancing, which he did. Several years later, my friend stated that he had never realized how much he had needed the physical contact that square dancing afforded him. He felt that the touching aspects of the dancing and the feeling of community had improved his health as much as, if not more than, the exercise from the dancing had. He wondered out loud if he could live without this important element in his life, and it seemed to me to be a very important question and one whose answer he knew. Most of us know the questions and the answers, but we do not know them apart from each other. They come into being through our meeting with each other, and this is the potential of the dialogical relationship.

Notes

1. Oliver Sacks, *The Man Who Mistook His Wife for a Hat and Other Clinical Tales* (New York: Harper and Row, 1987), p. xiii.
2. Ibid., p. 180.
3. Ibid., p. 186.
4. Garrett Porter & Patricia A. Norris, *Why Me? Harnessing the Healing Power of the Human Spirit* (New Hampshire: Stillpoint Publishing, 1985), p. 15.
5. Ibid., p. 9.
6. Ibid., pp. 28–29.
7. Ibid., pp. 28–29.
8. Ibid., p. 28.

CHAPTER 4

Pain As Touchstone of Reality

"Healing through meeting" is a phrase that was first introduced by Martin Buber and has subsequently been elaborated by Maurice Friedman. In this age of medical technology and advanced pharmacology the word "healing" has come to mean that which occurs when a therapeutic technique acts to reverse a particular pattern of illness. "Healing through meeting" emphasizes the healing that emanates from the healing partnership. When the patient is accepted as a partner, it is an act of confirmation. This act of confirmation arises from being present for the other, but does not imply that there is full mutuality within the partnership.

Disconfirmation most often arises out of early family relationships that deny the child confirmation in relation to his/her own uniqueness. The denial of confirmation causes a deep wound of the spirit and affects the whole being. Mistrust develops and one may feel unworthy of confirmation and/or mistrustful of those who attempt to confirm one in one's own uniqueness. To some extent, all therapists must deal with the effects of disconfirmation and the lack of trust that has grown out of early life experiences.

The first step in confirming the other is to establish a dialogue of touchstones.

> The real "dialogue of touchstones" means that we respond from
> where we are, and that we bring ourselves into the dialogue. The
> other person needs to know that he is really coming up against us
> as persons with touchstones and witnesses of our own.[1]

Some therapists find comfort in using certain techniques that
provide distance between the patient and the therapist. I have
known therapists who were very proud of their ability to confront
or to "shake up" their patients. There were times when the therapist appeared to be more interested in his/her performance than
the therapeutic process. There are also other, possibly more subtle,
ways of accomplishing distance.

When I first started working as a pain therapist I was given
two white laboratory coats. I was provided with laundry service
so that I would continue to have on hand a clean, starched, laboratory coat during my working hours. I felt that the coat was a
symbol of my professionalism and that I was now akin to all those
that donned these coats and walked our hallowed halls of healing.
To my credit I did not take on a professional tone of voice, for this
too serves to create a distance that makes it difficult to bring
oneself into the dialogue.

I was once part of a family therapy training group, where all
of the participants were professionals. Each of us shared aspects of
our own family history and others in the group responded. One
member shared a particularly painful aspect of her relationship
with her father, and another participant responded in a tone of
voice that was significantly different from her usual speaking
voice. She stated, "You are still angry at your father, aren't you?"
This simple statement/question and the change in her speaking
voice served to silence the other woman's voice. This was not
simply a question but was, by the very tone of the other's voice,
a judgment. The whole group was, to some extent, injured because
mistrust and caution diminished the potential for dialogue.

We all have various roles in life and there are expectations
that shape our behavior in each of these roles, but if we are to help
others establish a dialogue of touchstones we must bring ourselves into the dialogue. We cannot utilize the professional per-

sona to mask our own humanity. Doing so limits the potential for a healing partnership.

Both directly and indirectly, my own touchstones have opened the way toward meeting and confirming the other, and I, as therapist, try to provide for each patient an opening for a patient–therapist dialogue of touchstones. One touchstone for me is my initial encounter with psychotherapy. I was a third-year student at UCLA, and I was referred to the department of psychological services because of a psychosomatic disorder. My therapist was a young man who was serving as a psychiatric intern for one semester; I was a full-time student, the mother of two small children, and I was very disturbed about my marital situation. It was my first encounter with psychotherapy, and for many years this first experience would serve as my only frame of reference.

After a brief introductory session, the therapist administered several psychological tests. I remember wondering what he was testing for—what did he want to know about me? What would he learn about me that I did not know about myself? After the tests had been administered he invited me to talk about myself and my present concerns. I described my home life and situations that were causing extreme stress in my life. At one point the therapist stated that he could not believe that I was telling the truth. What I remember about this therapist is his hands. They were white, delicate, and very clean, and the nails were carefully manicured. They represented for me what I was unable to put into words but felt about his whole demeanor. I decided at that time that if I was to attain an improved state of health it would not and could not depend upon the help of this young man. We were close in age, but our worlds were distant and there was no way that he could imagine what was real for me.

At the end of the school year the therapist asked me if I would appear before a group of psychiatrists so that he could present my case history. In retrospect, I presume that it was a part of his internship requirement. I appeared, as requested, and the young psychiatrist and six other psychiatrists discussed my case. No one acknowledged my presence until I was called on to answer a few questions. I answered the questions, but I did not feel as though I had been heard. My own touchstones of reality were never revealed and the experience was not one of healing. The young psychiatrist had accomplished his own goals, but I was still wondering how any of this had addressed my own needs.

The patients I treat have usually been referred by a physician or a psychologist, but in some cases the patient is self-referred. Each patient brings his or her own expectations to this first meeting, and also brings not only present concerns, but a history that affects the present. From my own side, I have usually been able to review the patient's medical history, and it is here that serious illnesses, medications, and, possibly, psychological profiles are described. As an adjunct to the medical chart, I ask each patient to fill out a pain questionnaire that includes questions related to the patient's symptoms and current stressors. At this juncture, I know something about the patient, but I do not have a sense of the patient in his/her wholeness, as a unique person.

During the first session I begin to meet the patient, and it is through listening that I hear what is said, and through observing that I learn something about what is not said. Some patients are angry because they feel that they have been abandoned by their physician because they have failed to respond to medical treatment. Another patient may express skepticism, and feel that they are doomed to live in pain. Other patients want me to promise them that I can find a way to make them well, and in all cases, I begin to hear and observe the pain, fears, anger, and hope that each patient is expressing.

Sometimes, before the patient arrives, I want to resist being really present. There is a part of me that does not want to see beyond the medical descriptions of the patient, but I seldom feel this way once the patient has arrived. I begin to feel called upon by the other, and there is an unfolding that reveals the uniqueness of this person, who is also my patient. I am not aware of time, in the usual sense, and it is here that inclusion begins to take place. I do not mean to imply that, time after time, a predictable pattern occurs, but rather that what happens between us occurs despite my own resistances and/or effort to make it happen.

Karl

Karl was a 62-year-old man with essential hypertension and symptoms of stress. He took medications to control his hypertension, but the medications were becoming increasingly less effective. He had been hospitalized for one week, during the past year, for a complete medical evaluation. His medications were adjusted and a self-regulation program was suggested. The patient was referred for treatment and he was to monitor his blood pressure on a daily basis.

Karl completed the intake questionnaire and stated that he was most stressed by his symptoms and his spouse. He described himself as anxious, depressed, tense, energetic, and perfectionistic. I had read the medical chart, reviewed the intake questionnaire, and now Karl began to speak.

> I find it so hard to slow down. I feel like my body is running away with me. I've always been intense, and dedicated to my work, but now I fear that I may not be able to work if I can't keep my blood pressure under control.

Karl tended to speak very rapidly and he looked as though it was difficult for him to stay seated in his chair. I listened and responded, and then I asked him about his work.

> I am a civil servant and a volunteer chaplain. I consider my most important work that of being a chaplain. I work with male prisoners, at the county jail, and I was able to get this position through my job connections at the county offices. I am not financially able to retire, and anyway, I want to keep working or I might not be able to continue my work as a chaplain. My wife would like to see me retire, but I do not like the idea of being at home all day. She feels that I am away too much because of my extra work as a chaplain.

I asked Karl what he hoped to accomplish in the treatment program. "I hope to learn to control my high blood pressure and to feel less stressed."

This first treatment session lasted about 1½ hours. After a period of discussion, we moved to the lab, and I explained the relationship between hypertension and stress, and covered basic breathing techniques. This part of the session was somewhat routine, but it is within this context that a relationship begins to emerge. I sensed the patient's fears, but I waited for him to reveal what he felt comfortable expressing. We shared a small space and I tried to establish an opening without being intrusive. We needed to build a sense of trust and respect, and this is a delicate process. When the session ended, the patient was scheduled to come back in one week.

During each session we spent a period of our time talking and a period of time in the lab where Karl began to see how his emotions were affecting his physical state. We discussed his job, home life, and various other topics. I was aware of the importance of Karl's work as a chaplain, and one day we discussed why it was that being a chaplain was his avocation rather than his vocation. Karl's response to this question came from a position of trust.

> My earliest dreams were focused on being an Episcopalian priest. I was in my first year of training when the invasion of the German Army disrupted my studies. I was dedicated to nonviolence and had no intentions of entering into warfare, but the chain of circumstances changed my outlook. Until the invasion of my country I viewed the war from a distance, and I wanted to go on with my education and planned vocation. It wasn't just my own selfish desire to go on with my education; it was also my belief that taking another's life was wrong. I felt that I could not join forces to kill other human beings. This thinking preceded the invasion, of course, but my feelings about killing have never changed. The German Army took over our country, and they rounded up the Jews. It was not easy for any of us, but only the Jews faced almost certain death unless they could escape or hide out.
>
> I decided to join the resistance movement. Many of my friends had joined the movement, and I was young and wanted to make a

stand against the German invaders. It was a very dangerous business because we risked instant death if we were discovered, and
the raids could have easily ended up in costing us our lives. We
were not in the business of killing, but rather of destroying equipment and enemy supplies. Many of us were quite young and very
idealistic. I felt good about my participation in the resistance movement, but one night we were about to set off some explosives when
a couple of German soldiers appeared. We used the explosives to
kill them and I felt very responsible for the deaths of these two
soldiers. I did not quit the movement, and I know that other soldiers were killed during our maneuvers. I was aware that German
soldiers were killing off most of our Jewish population and they
would not have hesitated to kill me had they known about my
nighttime maneuvers. Still, I had vowed not to engage in killing,
and I now felt that I was unfit to become an Episcopalian priest. I
had defiled my dream by breaking my deepest conviction that I
should not kill other human beings.

At that point Karl paused. I knew that I had shared Karl's
deepest pain, his sorrow, and the guilt that he had borne over the
years. As mentioned earlier in this paper, inclusion is not a matter
of empathy or identification, but rather a bold swinging over to the
other's side. I stood my own ground, but that ground was somehow changed and I was more aware of my own humanity. This,
in part, explains my own period of resistance before the patient
arrives. I resist because I am not sure that I have the resources to
deal with what may be revealed by the patient, and I resist the
changes in my own ground that occur when I share the deepest
feelings of another. I saw this patient five years ago, and he remains a part of my being that continues to be shaped and reshaped
by the present.

If healing occurs, it arises from the between. There was nothing that I could say to assuage the pain and guilt that Karl felt, but
something did happen that had a healing effect. I think that the
patient felt confirmed as a person, and that this was the opening
way to a healing relationship. During the first few sessions of
therapy I do not, as a rule, confront the patient, or try to suggest
what might be causing the patient's symptoms. It is during these

first few sessions that a climate of trust is established and it is a time of listening.

Karl completed twelve sessions of biofeedback therapy and had a significant reduction in his blood-pressure level. A multidimensional approach was used, but at all times the dialogue was of great importance. There was a movement between the practical and the need to express feelings. The practical suggestions included breathing techniques, therapeutic walks, quieting exercises, speech-patterning suggestions, and discussions related to diet, exercise, and assertiveness. Deep abdominal breathing has a quieting effect on the whole body and a deep abdominal breath can be used to signal a relaxation response. A daily therapeutic walk affords a time to be present in the moment and to focus on what is present at that moment. Stretching exercises help to reduce chronic tension, and all types of exercise are very beneficial when developed in relation to individual needs. Yoga postures promote a quieting response as do certain other types of movement. Many individuals begin to speak very rapidly when they are stressed. Karl was chronically stressed and spoke rapidly, and his breathing pattern was shallow and irregular. Karl was encouraged to slow down his speech and to consciously pause, and take a breath after each sentence.

Karl needed to express his feelings in a less defensive way and this was discussed throughout the sessions. To build a climate of trust and improve communication between Karl and his wife we discussed what it means to listen to the other without feeling that we have to solve a problem or defend our own position. Karl had seldom shared his own fears with anyone and his wife did not understand why he did not want to retire. When he began to share some of his concerns with his wife, she became less insistent about his retirement. She had been very concerned about his health, and now felt less anxious since he was showing a marked improvement in terms of his blood pressure levels.

One of the main goals in the pain treatment program is to develop strategies that enable the patient to cope with the effects of stress and/or chronic pain. This reduces anxiety over the symptoms and encourages a caring attitude toward one's self rather than the feeling of victimization. The practical suggestions and the biofeedback readings helped Karl to understand how his whole body operated as a unit. He incorporated many of the suggestions into his daily life and he did improve. When last seen Karl was more relaxed, but aware that he needed to exercise a gentle vigilance in relation to his tendency to "go too fast."

Unless we live in a fairy tale world there is no possibility of living happily ever after. Karl will still have to deal with aging, retirement, unfulfilled dreams, and other life issues, but he was, when last seen, less anxious about his future, his health, and his relationship with his wife. We were both aware that each partnership has its limitations, but that we had made a reasonable amount of progress. From my own side I knew that I would never forget Karl, but I also knew that it was time for him to continue to work on his own. He knew that I cared about him and that I wished him well. Three months after our last session he sent me this poem and a short note about his continued progress.

Slow Me Down, Lord

Slow me down, Lord. Ease the pounding of my heart by the quieting of my mind. Steady my hurried pace with a vision of eternal reach of time.

Give me, amidst the confusion of my day, the calmness of the everlasting hills. Break the tensions of my nerves and muscles with the music of the singing streams that live in my memory.

Help me to know the magic restoring power of sleep.

Teach me the art of taking minute vacations . . . of slowing down to look at a flower, to chat with a friend, to pat a dog, to read a few lines from a good book.

Remind me each day of the fable of the hare and the tortoise that I may know that the race is not always to the swift; that there is more to life than increasing its speed.

Let me look upward into the branches of the towering oak and know that it grew great and strong because it grew slowly and well. Slow me down, Lord . . . and inspire me to send my roots deep into the soil of life's enduring values that I may grow toward the state of my own greater destiny.

Amen.

Wilfred A. Peterson

For some people pain becomes their main touchstone of reality. It becomes generalized and permeates every aspect of their life. The pain becomes a ruling force that dictates their every move. Some people become invalids and withdraw from family and friends. When a conversation does take place the pain takes center stage. People ask, "How is your pain today?" The person usually responds with an up-to-date pain report: "It's on the rampage today. It never leaves me for long, but today it hasn't let up. I can't move and I can't rest. The pain is killing me." This conversation may be repeated over and over again with minor changes in the inflection and content. It becomes an impersonal conversation, much as a discussion of the weather becomes somewhat routine and repetitive.

What happens to chronic-pain patients may also happen to persons with other chronic conditions. They may find that many people inquire about their health problems, but eventually it becomes little more than a polite inquiry. How is your asthma? How have your allergies been? Have those ulcers settled down? There is little room for dialogue if a chronic condition takes over one's identity. It then becomes their only touchstone of reality.

Cancer and other catastrophic diseases can also become chronic conditions. The initial concern for the individual gives way to an uncomfortable silence or brief inquiries that elude the life-and-death struggle that the person may be going through. When one becomes wedded to one's disease and/or pain there is a loss of personhood. The will to live is often diminished and one is consumed from within. It is a self-destructive course that is often fostered by family members and friends.

If the patient's touchstone of reality is his or her pain then it must be acknowledged before they can begin to gain a sense of self beyond the pain. This occurs when there is a shift in the treatment protocol. The patient is brought into a partnership of healing that strengthens his or her resources and serves to enhance his or her self-regulation skills. This is best accomplished in a supportive treatment program that offers a multidimensional approach that includes both medical and nonmedical modalities. All too often the patient is not referred for pain therapy until all of the various medical modalities have been exhausted.

The longer a patient has suffered from chronic pain or other chronic symptoms the more difficult it is to treat. Many patients have endured years of pain and disappointment. There may be a history of failed surgeries, medication abuse, "doctor shopping," excessive wear and tear on one or more body parts, emotional and/or physical traumas, or any number of other causes, but once the problem becomes a chronic disorder most people find themselves deserted in a medical wasteland. By this time the patient has often incorporated the pain into the very core of their being and it has permeated every aspect of their life. The patient is gradually consumed by his or her pain, and feelings of anger, futility, and despair exacerbate the symptoms.

Excellent pain treatment programs are available, but they are usually quite costly and are not accessible to the majority of the population. I usually recommend that the patient seek out a support system that will help to enhance my own treatment structure. Most patients that I see receive ongoing medical treatment, individual psychotherapy, and/or group psychotherapy as well as pain therapy. Massage, yoga, dance therapy, physical therapy, acupuncture, and chiropractic treatments are only a few of the modalities that may serve to help the patient to ease their pain. It is important for patients to participate in the healing process by making choices, and to realize that seldom does one modality serve to change a complex condition like chronic pain. It is also important for the patient to realize that he or she has the right to be treated with respect and to be heard.

Julie

Julie had forgotten what a day without pain and breathing difficulty was like. She arrived at the office looking tired and despondent. She stated that she had a headache and neck and shoulder pain and that she was having some difficulty speaking and breathing. She explained that sometimes she would be talking on the telephone and her voice would just "give out." I did not rush her and she was able to talk about her symptoms and how they had begun. Julie's medical chart included a patient history, but it is important to hear this information from the patient's perspective. Julie spoke softly, but clearly.

> My whole life has changed. I used to work, participate in activities with my children, lead an active life with my husband, and feel good about myself. In the last six months my health has deteriorated and so has everything else in my life. I have gained about thirty pounds and I feel like a slug. Most of the time I am fatigued and I barely complete my basic household chores.

Julie went on to explain how she had been exposed to some toxic fumes.

> One morning, I went to work, as usual, and I was feeling fine. About two hours later I started feeling like I was coming down with a cold or something. My eyes were watering, my nose and throat began to hurt and I began to cough. Several other employees began to have similar symptoms, but before we had a chance to question what was going on the supervisor arrived. She stated that some fumes had been accidentally released through the office ventilation system and that we would be given the day off. We were told that the situation was a temporary one and that the nurse was available if we were feeling ill. I had no idea what type of fumes I had been exposed to or how this had happened. I did not go to the nurse because I wanted to get out of the building as soon as possible. That evening I still had some eye irritation and I coughed off and on. The next day I had a slight headache and mild symptoms, but I returned to my workplace. Our supervisor assured us that the problem had been cleared up. Several hours later my head was

"pounding" and I was having some difficulty breathing. My desk was very close to the vent and I wondered if I had inhaled more of the fumes than the others had. I told my supervisor that I needed to see the nurse. I was examined by the company nurse and she could find no visible signs of upper respiratory irritation. She wondered if my present illness was coincidental with the release of the fumes. I was on and off of the job for a few weeks and then I just took off of work. I was sent to a company doctor and he gave me a prescription for some medication and an inhaler. I think that he thought that I was exaggerating my discomfort, but he didn't have to live with my symptoms. The medication has helped me, but I have become very dependent on the inhaler. I haven't returned to work because I am afraid that I will just get worse again.

Julie had been off work for over six months and she had only received minimal medical treatment. The company doctor saw her once a month and he checked her response to the medications and encouraged her to consider going back to work. Julie was very upset by his lack of concern.

I am beginning to wonder if I will ever be able to breathe without an inhaler. I know that I am not extremely ill, but I'm not well either; I am fatigued, I have headaches, I lose my voice, my breathing is not normal, my throat is often sore, my neck muscles are tense, I have difficulty sleeping and most of all I am afraid of what is happening to me.

Life beyond her symptoms had begun to fade for Julie. She had a loving family and they were supportive of her, but a chronic condition stresses every member of the family. Her symptoms were a constant reminder of the family's inability to relieve her pain and discomfort. A chronic condition becomes a burden to be borne by the whole family. There was also anger and frustration, and this led to feelings of guilt. How can one justify being angry at someone who is suffering?

Julie was not the same person that her family had known and loved. They still loved her, but they missed the person that had been able to work outside of her home and still had enough energy to care for and enjoy her family. They also missed the economic gains that her working had afforded them. Now she was off of work and she had barely enough energy to take care of herself. They had expected her to get well and to return to work, but she seemed to be getting worse. Julie was focused on her symptoms and she showed little interest in the day-to-day concerns and activities of her family.

Julie's family began to re-group and she became less of a participant and more of an observer. She seldom voiced her opinions and was left out of the family's decision-making process. Few families have the resources to give the support and guidance that a person with chronic pain and/or a chronic condition needs. Julie was losing her personhood and she needed professional help to regain her sense of self.

Patients that have been emotionally and/or physically injured on the job often feel that once they are away from their workplace they will begin to feel better, but this seldom occurs. Julie had received only minimal health care and she had only her family to turn to, and this was not enough. In the months following her injury her symptoms grew progressively worse and were exacerbated by her emotional distress. Once she was in a supportive program, however, she did begin to improve. Before seeing me she was evaluated by a psychiatrist, had a psychological interview, and was placed in a group therapy program with other patients who suffered from chronic pain and/or a chronic condition. The patients in this group had also been injured at their workplace.

Once Julie realized that her symptoms were being taken seriously and that she was being heard, it was easier to introduce ways to help her to help herself. We moved between self-regulation strategies and ways to give her back her voice, both literally and figuratively. Julie was aware of increased neck tension before her voice began to fade, but she was not aware of the changes in her breathing patterns. I utilized EMG biofeedback to help her decrease the muscle tension in her neck and shoulders and we worked on relaxed breathing. Julie was taught to take a breath from the diaphragm and she began to recognize and change her habit of "shallow" breathing. This too contributed to lessening her chronic neck and shoulder tension.

The therapist may have an excellent treatment plan, but there must be room for flexibility. Patient setbacks and unexpected events may demand a different approach. The patient's tempo is important and the challenge of adjustment should be borne by the therapist. It is not healthy for the patient to feel that he/she needs to meet the expectations of the therapist. Julie was motivated and sensitive to her own needs. This helped me to plan a more effective treatment and to allow for necessary changes along the way. I introduced the various biofeedback modalities and I also emphasized the need to learn to utilize these skills throughout the day. Julie's fatigue had lingered on and I asked her what she did when she was feeling less fatigued. "When I am feeling pretty good I try to do things around the house. I never catch up and I feel guilty if I feel good and just sit around."

This common problem afflicts most chronic-pain patients. Instead of reinforcing their decreased symptoms they hurry to take unfair advantage of their improved state. It is important for a patient to realize that they are not wasting time when they take time to reinforce a period of decreased symptoms. They are doing the important work of reestablishing an image of wellness. This does not mean that all tasks must be set aside, but it does mean that reasonable limits need to be set. This also serves to establish a sense of self-worth and control over one's own symptoms.

One way that I measured Julie's progress was her change of focus. She began to express her plans for the future and to take more interest in her family. I had encouraged Julie to insist upon a more complete medical diagnosis, and we had often discussed possibilities. One week she announced that she had taken a very decisive step toward circumventing her company's medical treatment policy. This was a major breakthrough and I knew that she was beginning to find her own voice. She still had her symptoms but they were no longer crowding out the other aspects of her life. She continued to have what she called "bad periods of pain and gloom," but she knew that she had gotten through some very difficult periods and this gave her strength. She had more confidence in herself and she had a wider circle of support. Our touchstones of reality come into being as we struggle to confront the events of our life and to bear witness to them, without losing a sense of our own personhood in relation to the event.

Note

1. Maurice Friedman, *The Healing Dialogue in Psychotherapy* (New York: Jason Aronson, 1985), p. 207.

CHAPTER 5

Distance and Relation and the Development of the Person

It is my basic premise that "healing through meeting" is a viable, dynamic component of the healing process. In order to understand the full impact of this statement it is important to determine what it means to be human. Becoming a human being is a process of growth and this growth must be nurtured by other human beings. We are not solitary creatures; we come into being in relation to others and it is in relation to others that we learn what it means to be fully human. The basic principle here relates to the writings of Martin Buber and Maurice Friedman and concerns the concept of distance and relation.

At its beginning, human life has much in common with that of all living creatures. There is a sense of oneness with all that comes into one's realm of being and heightened sensory awareness. The human baby, like other living creatures, does not have a sense of self and does not recognize the otherness of those that seek to meet its needs. What is unique about human life is the ability to see beyond the immediate environment and to develop a self through the twofold movements of distancing and relation.

As the infant moves from a state of unity to the primal setting at a distance there is a growing sense that the other being is different from and looms over against him/her. This is a gradual movement that begins between the infant and its mother and relates to being called into existence.

Being called into existence is related to each person's need for confirmation. Human life cannot exist without some measure of confirmation, and to become fully human we need to be able to both receive and to give confirmation to others. Babies and all small children need to be called into existence as persons and to be confirmed in their uniqueness as the persons that they are and in what they may become and are called to become. As Maurice Friedman points out, "basic confirmation gives us our ticket to exist and the confirmation along the road has to do with the way in which we exist." Martin Buber states:

> Sent forth from the natural domain of species into the hazard of the solitary category, surrounded by the air of a chaos which came into being with him, secretly and bashfully he watches for a Yes which allows him to be and which can come to him only from one human person to another. It is from one man to another that the heavenly bread of self-being is passed.[1]

Genuine relation between persons means acceptance of otherness. The other is confirmed in his/her being. Without genuine meeting man/woman cannot confirm the other. Relation can only occur when we are fully present to another, and in the making oneself present to another one is made present to his/her self by the other, "together with mutuality of acceptance, of affirmation and confirmation."

To be denied basic confirmation from a significant other during childhood may create a vacuum within that can never be filled and will, as mentioned earlier, affect one's ability to give and receive confirmation. One is, in a sense, given no ground of his or her own and what ground he/she has is, at best, shaky. The child who is denied confirmation from the significant other may begin to believe that nothing good can happen to him/her and he/she does not deserve to have more than the crumbs of life to call his or her own.

The child who is denied his or her own ground has great difficulty holding onto the ground that he or she does have and takes on a feeling of guilt. He or she sees him- or herself as undeserving of love and to be blamed for being unlovable. He or she feels guilty of a crime that he or she cannot identify, and his or her mistrust and self-denial serves to cut him or her off from the very world that is needed for the development of a self. The self, in order to know itself as an I, needs the world and those who dwell in the world so that it may know what it means to be whole. The confirmation that we seek can only be attained through real meeting, but, as Maurice Friedman has pointed out, too often the dialogue is used as a means to an end, and one's own uniqueness, as well as the other's, is lost. The other is treated as "an object to be known and used."

When persons are not confirmed in their uniqueness they may settle for what Maurice Friedman refers to as the "contract"—"confirmation with strings attached." This confirmation may be very positive, but there is an invisible contract. The contract usually starts in childhood and states that being a good child or acting in some particular way will gain confirmation. "Being good" extends into the adult years, but now being good may mean fulfilling a particular economic role or the bringing of prestige to the family name. One is not confirmed for his/her own uniqueness, but for the role that he/she maintains. This is carried beyond the family to the community. The doctor, for example, may be confirmed not as a person, but as a doctor. The true paradox of confirmation is that the person cannot develop an "I" without the social, but he/she cannot develop an "I" by remaining only in the social. There must be a tension between the two and then the person must hold this tension throughout his or her life. Few people are completely successful in maintaining this tension.

> Everybody must play a social role, as a means to economic livelihood and as the simplest prerequisite for any sort of relations with other people in the family and society. On the other hand, one cannot resolve the tension by sacrificing personal confirmation; for this suppression of a basic human need results in an anxiety that

may be more and more difficult to handle as the gap between person and role widens. To stand in this tension, however, is to insist that one's confirmation in society also be in some significant sense a confirmation of oneself as a unique person who does not fit into any social category.[2]

The "Yes" that each infant awaits is the call to existence, and it is related to basic confirmation. The first days, months, and years of one's life establish the foundation for additional confirmation. When basic confirmation is lacking, a child suffers, and this suffering not only affects its basic humanity, but relates to lifelong patterns of health. What we commonly refer to as stress-related chronic pain disorders are frequently best described as disorders of relationship. Each person must be called into this world by another, and at all times we exist in relationship. Without genuine meeting between persons the quality of life is diminished and a degree of pain, suffering, and stress is a consequence. What may be the greatest paradox of confirmation is the fact that what is needed most to sustain the quality of life cannot be willed and the emptiness within may be the driving force that creates increased tension and stress as one seeks to fill this empty vacuum.

The early dialogue is vital to our health and influences our ability to go out into the world and establish relationships with other beings. We need the unconditional love that originates from our sense of oneness with the mother, and we also need the personal wholeness that comes from our achievement of separateness. Kaplan calls this our "second birth"; it is a continuing lifelong task.

> Our adult actions are but distant echoes, reflections, metaphorical paraphrases of the events of our second birth. Even so, adulthood is not the end of childhood or the completion of a journey that goes only forward. The maturing adult is continually reliving and revising his memories of childhood, refining his identity, reforging the shape of his selfhood, discovering new facets of his being.[3]

The choreography of our whole life is colored by the relationships and events of our early life. We carry into the present that which has been part of our past and the wounds and injuries of our early life affect present relationships and the state of our health. Then too there is tragedy. It may enter our life at any time and affect the strength of our being.

> ... sometimes fortune is too harsh for even the most courageous and firmly rooted. There are letdowns that are unbearable; a home swept away by a fire or hurricane, forced retirement from a lifelong job, the desertion of a loved one, the stillborn baby, the death of a child or a parent. When disaster strikes, the absence of community that is typical in our alienating contemporary societies leaves us totally vulnerable and unprepared.[4]

Many patients express feelings of pain and sorrow that relate to early disconfirmation. Jean was one such patient and while the disconfirmation was not a source of her pain, it was an underlying source of her inability to manage her pain. She was referred for pain therapy two years after an initial back injury. Surgical intervention was not indicated, and pain medications were no longer satisfactory for management of the pain.

Jean was 59 years old and worked full time as a payroll clerk. Her greatest fear, she stated, was being unable to work, as she needed her full income to manage her household expenses. She filled out a pain questionnaire and we discussed her answers. She had daily lower back pain that worsened throughout the workday. She found it difficult to relax after work and had multiple symptoms of chronic stress. The symptoms included sleep disturbance, overeating, neck and shoulder tension, and fatigue.

In time Jean shared the fact that she was twice divorced and had one daughter and two grandsons. She saw her daughter only when she initiated the visit, and her grandsons were now teenagers and "constantly on the go." She occasionally saw them, but it was mainly when they were rushing to go somewhere with only enough time for a quick hello. She stated that she had seen her daughter and grandchildren more frequently when her services as a "babysitter" had been needed.

Jean had gained weight after her injury and she was self-conscious about her current weight. She stated that her former husband had been eight years younger than she and that they had enjoyed an active life together, but one year after the injury he "walked out on me. I think that he was afraid that he would have to take care of me." Jean had one sister, but they were not close. She stated that her sister was well off and happily married. "We talk now and then by telephone, but I get the feeling that she does not want a third party hanging around." She had friends at work and one friend outside of her workplace that she had not called for over a month. She enjoyed being at home and often worked on craft projects.

During our initial sessions of pain therapy we worked on pain-management strategies. Jean learned to become more aware of the subtle signs of increasing tension. She was able to decrease her symptoms with a "signal breath," tense-relax exercises, and calming affirmations. She decreased unnecessary tasks and began to take short breaks for relaxation practice. Through these practical applications of her pain therapy program she began to gain confidence in her ability to manage her own symptoms. During each session there was ample time for Jean's own voice, and it is here that the unfolding of her own resources came into being.

Around the fourth or fifth session of pain therapy Jean stated:

> I always felt unwanted by my mother. She called me my father's child, and she was critical and abusive from the time of my birth. My sister, who was born three years later, was treated well in contrast and was seldom scolded. My father worked out of town and was seldom at home. When he was at home, he would try to protect me from my mother's anger. I was sure that my mother disliked me because I was a disappointment to her. I was tall, thin, and clumsy and she was often critical of my appearance. My parents never divorced, but my father's periods of absence and his support of me were endless sources of my mother's anger. When I was about eighteen, I learned that my mother had been pregnant with me before her marriage to my father. Being part of a small community she had inflicted shame not only on herself but on her

whole family. My grandparents showed no fondness for my father, and there was never a closeness between our family and my mother's family, or for that matter with my father's family either. Now I knew why my mother referred to me as my father's child. I understood why she seemed to resent me. But I have never really healed. My father died while I was still in my twenties, and my mother lived on for another fifteen years. She remained critical of me and of my husband, and she was not close to my daughter.

We discussed what had given her strength over the years and also what was helping her at this time. One thing that helped her to relax was the use of relaxation tapes. I had given her several for home use, and I sometimes introduced a new tape during the pain therapy session. On one such occasion, I utilized a visual imagery tape that was designed to guide her through a beautiful garden with childlike appreciation. Jean loved plants and had a small garden that she tended at her home. The session seemed to be going well and then she began to sob. I became frightened by this sudden outburst of emotion and I stopped the tape. I asked her if she was alright and if the tape had made her sad. She stopped crying and stated that she was not sad. "The garden was beautiful and there on a bench was my father. He looked handsome and he smiled at me. I was like a child and I felt shy. I did not move, but I cried because I was so happy to see him." I felt that my own fears had interrupted a beautiful moment for Jean, but she did not complain. She asked if she could use the tape at home, and she reassured me that she viewed her experience as a very positive one. Jean was also receiving group therapy so I encouraged her to discuss her experience with her therapist, if she felt the need to do so. Jean left the office stating that it had been an important session for her, and I remained there with lingering doubts about her using the tape in an unsupported environment and about my need to interrupt her during the session.

The next week Jean came into the session and was eager to tell me what had happened when she had used the tape at home. She had once again entered the garden as part of the guided imagery, but this time she was an adult and her father greeted her from the path. Again he smiled at her, but this time he also spoke to her and said, "I love you." Jean had tears in her eyes, but she seemed relaxed and calm. "I have always doubted that my father could love me now that I am older and less attractive. I feel now that he does still love me and I will always remember that."

What I learn, time and time again, is that healing is not just a matter of science and technology. There is a personal aspect of healing that cannot be replicated. Jean continued to improve over the next few months. She used all of her home practice tapes, but the garden tape remained her favorite one. The meeting with her father did not occur again, and she did not lament its passing but rather treasured what had happened. She seemed confirmed by her experience and more at peace with herself. Her pain management skills were vastly improved, and she had more confidence in her own abilities to apply the pain management skills as needed. She also knew when to ask for help.

It is important for the patient to rebuild, or in some cases, to begin to build a community where full mutuality is possible. I encouraged Jean to strengthen her relationship with her daughter and to initiate a simple activity with the friend she had not been in touch with for some time. I tapered off the frequency of our sessions and moved toward a termination date. There would be a post-period that would be open to her, if additional sessions were needed.

All relationships test the limits of mutuality. Jean was beginning to successfully rebuild her own community and to partake in the give and take of these relationships. She had tended to underestimate her own resources. During the pain therapy sessions she had learned to decrease her symptoms and she had also gained a better sense of herself. From the beginning I was struck by her outgoing, friendly personality, her use of color and how it enhanced her appearance, and her courage as she continued to work despite her discomfort. She was very modest. Her many years of disconfirmation made it difficult to accept confirmation but she was learning to do so. Saying goodbye to a patient is a "vote of confidence," but may also be painful. There is at times a desire to sustain and support the patient, but this would satisfy my needs not the patient's needs. I knew that it was time to let go and so did Jean.

Each patient tests, to some degree, the limits of the helper's responsibility to the patient. Every patient does not get well, and loneliness, a lifetime of disconfirmation, and/or tragedy are all realities that cannot be erased or reversed. It may be difficult for the therapist to set limits on his or her own efforts to help "make" the patient well, and the patient may feel that he/she must show some improvement in order to please the therapist. Then too, there are limits related to availability of time and personal resources. It is doubtful that any one person can make up for another person's lack of parenting or years of disconfirmation, but it is possible for some healing to occur when "healing through meeting" takes place.

My own limits of responsibility were tested, not by a patient, but by a friend. When I first met Anne she was a successful teacher, the mother of two bright children, and had a lovely home. I mainly knew her from a distance because we had a mutual friend, and I mainly took the role of admiring this woman who appeared to have attained so much of what I hoped to attain in my own life. These first brief meetings occurred over 30 years ago and I could not have imagined, at that time, how troubled and angry this seemingly successful woman was.

Anne was one of three children born to an affluent family in the early 1920s. Her father was a respected scientist and the owner of a successful manufacturing company. Her mother had been a teacher before her marriage, but had not worked outside of the home since the marriage. Anne was the middle child, and she felt that her older brother was her mother's favorite child and that her younger sister was her father's favorite child. When discussing her family, she would say that she was liked by her childless aunt, but was, otherwise, the outsider in her family. She was gifted musically and artistically and did well at school. Anne's brother and sister were both artistic and musically inclined, but they were also highly gifted in science and math. Anne's father, by obtaining the results of school intelligence tests, had informed each child of their standing in the family. Anne's brother was the most intelligent, her sister was a close second, and Anne was in third place.

Anne's brother was restless and belligerent. He did not finish high school, joined the Navy and later married a woman who did not meet his family's standards. When he was about 25 years old and struggling to support his family, his father offered him a place in the company, which he accepted, and he eventually inherited the company from his father. Anne's sister completed one year of college and then went to work at a department store. She married a Bohemian artist and was, to some extent, partially supported by her father until his death. Anne completed her college degree, became a teacher, married the man that her parents most approved of and was financially independent. What she did not attain was the unconditional love of her parents, and her anger and frustration became the tools of self-destruction.

Fifteen years after my first brief meetings with Anne we began to form a friendship. By this time Anne, our mutual friend, and I were all divorced, and had, between us, eight children to care for. We all moved into a large house and set up a communal household. Each evening Anne would start to drink, and by bedtime she was inebriated and emotionally upset. During these times she would curl up and cry herself to sleep. The only part of Anne's life that seemed to have stayed intact was her teaching position, but, in time, this too would fall apart.

I lived with Anne and our mutual friend for two years, and I shared Anne's pain on a daily basis. I also shared the pleasures of a close and loving friendship, but I could never begin to fill the void that had been created by her lack of early confirmation. Anne found it difficult to look at herself in the mirror and stated that she had always felt very uncomfortable when she was faced with her own image.

I often think of my own early images of Anne. She was attractive, appeared to be confident, and seemed to have such a beautiful home and family. I was not aware of the fact that Anne detested her husband and avoided him through her drinking and frequent trips away from home. Her husband, who was greatly admired by the family, had severe problems that were well hidden from all but his most intimate family members. One year after Anne divorced her husband he was killed, and while not involved she still felt guilty about having left him.

During the two years that I lived with Anne, unbeknownst to me at the time, she became my teacher. She shared what it meant to be unconfirmed and to suffer from the pain of existential guilt. I learned that her own personal truth had little relationship to the personal truth of her family of origin. When she would express feelings to a family member, that person would attempt to correct her "incorrect perceptions," and this would serve to further erode her right to exist as a worthwhile person. I learned that a person can be very disturbed and still have the resources to give to others. Anne was a fine teacher, she was a loyal friend, and she shared her love of music and her hospitality with both friends and family. She also helped to heal her own family and to restore trust and love within her immediate family. All this was accomplished, however, despite the fact that she herself remained a very wounded human being. I loved Anne, and I valued her friendship, but I learned that I did not have the resources to heal her wounds, and that, without limits, her needs could become all consuming. When she cried herself to sleep at night, she was remembering and experiencing the void within that had existed since her birth. This void increased over the years and Anne became, I feel, more and more vulnerable to both her internal world and to the external world that had never really called her into being.

I visited Anne after a prolonged illness on her part. She was lying in a hospital bed, in the home where she had grown up. It was now her daughter's home, but she had a bedroom upstairs, and all around her were reminders of her childhood. I greeted her, and then I spoke to other family members. She turned her face to the wall, and I knew that she was unhappy about my lack of attention. In time, I pulled up a chair, and we spoke. She was in pain and it was hard for her to say much, but I held her hand and stroked her head. She told me that she wanted to stay at home and that she was afraid to go to the hospital. She had been in and out of the hospital during the past year and feared that she would not be strong enough to come home again. Much of our time together was spent in gentle silence, but one of the last things that Anne said to me was, "I feel like my heart is bleeding."

Anne was taken to the hospital on the day following our visit. Many tests were taken, and it was determined that she was in the advanced stages of cancer. She had been in and out of hospitals during the past year because of a stroke and an injury to her leg, but cancer had not been detected during this time. Her family called me and told me that she was "failing fast" and that she was no longer coherent. When I saw Anne again, it was exactly seven days after our previous visit. She was tied down and was thrashing in her bed. She had refused to eat, and food tubes were in her nose. When she saw me, she told me that they had hurt her and that she wanted me to take her home. She then went on to say that she knew that I wouldn't help her, and she cursed and vented her anger. Her eyes were glazed and she did not seem to know that it was me, but she did know that someone had entered the room. I had been told that she said the same thing to everyone, but that she became especially violent if she heard certain family voices. I felt that she had been violated, and was, in a sense, being tortured. I could feel the anger of a lifetime being vented on everyone who viewed her state but could offer no relief. It was the final insult, and she somehow managed to express the rage that she had usually vented on herself.

I saw Anne one more time before she died. Her family had wanted her moved to the hospice, but her violent behavior was preventing this. The hospice staff decided that they would accept her, and she was moved into this loving environment about ten days before she died. The hospice staff exemplified what is meant by the term "healing through meeting." They were caring and respected Anne's humanity. She was no longer violent and she was able to sip the malts that they provided. When I last saw her, she was resting comfortably. Three days later she stopped breathing and quietly died.

A memorial service was held for Anne, and her junior high school science teacher and long-time family friend sang two of her favorite hymns. Then this 85-year-old man reminisced about the 13-year-old Anne. He remembered her as a lovely, bright, and joyful student. She was this and more, but she never believed that it was so. Anne taught me that the wounds of childhood may remain dormant for years, but that they never disappear. I have spoken with 80-year-old patients who are in physical pain, and they often speak of their early traumas as the greatest pain that they have ever suffered. When "healing through meeting" occurs there is healing, yet, as in the case of Anne, it is not necessarily a healing of the body, but rather a healing of the spirit. It is the kind of healing that enables the person to utilize their own resources to reestablish a healing dialogue with their family, their community, and with their own being. It may also be the kind of healing that enables one to die in peace and with dignity. The movement is toward a climate of trust and toward reaching out and touching the other. It is a movement toward a community that allows room for each person to have a ground of his or her own and a voice that expresses his or her own uniqueness. Maurice Friedman points out:

> The helpfulness of the therapist does not lie in the fact that he or she is a better Socratic dialectician or that he or she articulates better, but rather that he or she can help the patient out of the unfruitful either/or of choosing between faithfulness to one's own emergent touchstones and relation with the community. Yet this is only possible in a situation of mutual trust. If the patient fears to expose himself for fear that the therapist or the family or his friends will invalidate what he has to contribute as worthless, then he will not be able to enter into a dialogue of touchstones. The goal of healing through meeting, of confirmation, and of the dialogue of touchstones is, therefore, the same—to establish a dialogue on the basis of trust. There is something the patient brings that no one else in the world can—his uniqueness.[5]

Notes

1. Martin Buber, *The Knowledge of Man: A Philosophy of The Interhuman,* edited with an introduction by Maurice Friedman (New York: Harper and Row, 1966), p. 71.
2. Maurice Friedman, *The Confirmation of Otherness in Family, Community and Society* (New York: Pilgrim Press, 1983), pp. 56–57.
3. Louise G. Kaplan, *Oneness and Separateness: From Infant to Individual* (New York: Simon and Schuster, 1978), p. 32.
4. Ibid., pp. 44–45.
5. Maurice Friedman, *The Healing Dialogue in Psychotherapy* (New York: Jason Aronson, 1985), p. 218.

CHAPTER 6

Stress, Willfulness, and the Decline of the Healing Dialogue

It is the family and the community that generally offer the confirmation that each individual must have in order to become fully human. When the family and community are no longer a stable force within the society, the much-needed confirmation may be lacking and even within the family one may feel abandoned and lonely. When one is given very little confirmation, there are signs of this deprivation at every stage of one's life. This lack of confirmation often drives one to attempt to will what cannot be willed. This is part of the web of desperation that actually prevents the attainment of confirmation and prevents the dialogue of caring and loving from taking place.

In his book *The Ways of The Will,* Leslie Farber describes the will as "the mover of actions both trivial and important." He sees the will as emanating from two different realms. The first realm is that which occurs without our making the conscious effort to make it happen, and the second realm dwells in the conscious state of thinking where we knowingly will a particular action to take place. The will of the first realm is what we might think of as "flow." It is that which moves naturally into being and is to be

71

found in the graceful movements of a dancer, the silence between friends or lovers, the tenderness of a loving mother, the spontaneous laughter of children, and unfolding of a flower. We are at these moments "of a piece—mind and body seamlessly and unself-consciously joined in a totality." The will is a part of the action, but it is so much a part of our faculties that we are not consciously planning each new move; our efforts seem to be effortless.

In the first realm of the will there is movement in a direction, but not toward a particular object.

> Direction, here, is to be understood not as an ideal goal toward which we press, however much we falter, but rather as a way interspersed with, yet not obstructed by, worldly detail and worldly objectives. Direction, therefore, is a way whose end cannot be known—a way open to possibility, including the possibility of failure.[1]

This is not a realm where human relations must occur, but the dialogic potentiality is to be found here. This is a realm of freedom; the freedom to speak forthrightly and to do so even though the hazards of doing so may be obvious. You might say that in the first realm the self is not the dominant focus, but the expression of the will flows in a way that leads one in a direction that reveals the self as no other movement could.

Farber describes the will of the second realm as a utilitarian will. Here a person is seen as moving toward a particular object rather than in a direction. There is usually a conscious willing to see something accomplished and there is an absorption that makes one much less available to the possibility of relation.

In the will of the first realm there is flow, but this does not imply that the results are always satisfactory. In the will of the second realm we can separate and examine what we are doing and what it is that we want to do. Farber states that

> All of us . . . live our lives in both realms, trusting that the achievements of the second realm will correct the indulgences of the first, and that the freedom of the first realm will provide some direction and scope for the activity of the second.[2]

We need the second realm for our everyday life. Much of our education is accomplished here and this is the realm where technological advances occur, but, as Farber states, it is here too that the disordered will occurs when the will of the second realm tries to do the work of the will of the first realm.

> ... increasingly we apply the will of the second realm to those portions of life that not only will not comply, but that become distorted—even vanish—under coercion.[3]

Farber points out that this seems to be "The Age of the Disordered Will." We are enslaved by our desire to will what cannot be willed. There are portions of our lives that will not comply with the will, and the disordered will results from using the will of the second realm in a willful way. We will to will and the result is anxiety.

This is a time when we are often led to believe that we can control every aspect of our life. We are told that we should be able to will ourselves to sleep, will ourselves to a healthful state, will a meaningful relationship, and will away the anxiety that results from this extreme willfulness. The media promotes a multitude of products that promise to produce a life where one is wholly subject to will. The media have promoted aspirin, laxatives, and other products to help dispel our miseries, and the professionals have built up their business with the promises of tranquilizers, stimulants, psychoanalysis, sleeping pills, and various "how to" books and classes. When we try to will what cannot be willed, anxiety is likely to occur and this is seen as an ache that helplessly cries for relief. The result is a split between the will and its object and finally a split between the body and the mind.

We do not have to look far to see examples of the will attempting to will what cannot be willed. Whenever a person's world is threatened, in any way, there is a reaction that reflects something about who and where that person is in his/her world. The person may display grief, despair, or remorse, but anxiety will not appear until he/she uses his will to counter the threat and to attempt to will what cannot be willed. The will stubbornly pursues a particular object and reason, imagination, and the like are diminished.

The ability to objectify, diversify, or to dispel is lost and the result is that the will/object split widens and as this occurs the body/mind split also begins to widen.

Adults, as well as young people, are developing an ever-increasing dependence on drugs and it is a major problem within our society. Leslie Farber illuminates the multiple uses of drugs on every level of our society.

> Drugs are used to relieve anxiety, but more than this, they tend to give the "illusion of healing the split between the will and its refractory object."
>
> The resulting feeling of wholeness may not be a responsible one, but at least within that wholeness—no matter how willful the drugged state may appear to an outsider—there seems to be, briefly and subjectively, a responsible and vigorous will. This is the reason, I believe, that the addictive possibilities of our age are so enormous.[4]

There is, Farber believes, a real hunger for a sovereign and irreducible will; one that is so wedded to our reason, imagination, and intentions that we are not even aware of its presence. This is the flow or direction that one takes as opposed to the movement toward a particular objective. This is not to say that we can ever remain in a state of flow, but when there is harmony between the realm of the first will and the realm of the second will, there is unity in one's state of being and freedom from the bondage that occurs when one is driven by an isolated will.

When we dwell in the will of the second realm there comes a time when there is a loss that is, at times, felt in the deepest way, but there is also an ongoing effort to keep up our willful pace and to never stop long enough to see where we have been, where we are, and where we are going. The split that Farber describes widens, and we are cut off and isolated from our own wholeness and relation with others. We stand alone and yet the frantic pace of the realm of the disordered will offers the illusion that this is not so, and we keep attempting to will that which cannot be willed.

The will of the second realm has helped the countries of the

Western world to become the most technologically advanced in the world, but when this will is applied to the will of the first realm we see the effects of the disordered will. The mind/body split serves to drive us on toward the impossible goal of controlling both the world that we live in and of overcoming all obstacles of our own being. The cost of this impossible goal is anxiety, stress, and stress-related disorders that often lead to pain, illness, and premature death. Brown states:

> In his physical dimensions man is a full foot taller than he was last century. In the confusion of a rapidly expanded material life it was to be expected that growth of the mind would be more difficult to recognize, perhaps more difficult to realize. Today the world is filled with signs of an approaching era of extended mental abilities. It may be that a first step toward realizing these is becoming aware that the failure of minds to achieve a world of harmony is because they have been diverted from an original purpose of knowing the harmony between mind and body.[5]

The split between the mind and body occurs when we live in the world of objects—when we see the world as distanced from ourselves and begin to seek our confirmation by manipulation and/or appearing to be what we believe others want us to be. Here the ground does not support us and we tend to cling desperately to what ground we have. The disordered will takes over and the illusion of wholeness may be gained through alcohol and drugs. There is a frantic effort to gain control over the environment and a sense of loss that cannot be identified. Relation is lost and with it the confirmation that we so desperately need. The flow that is identified with the will of the first realm is denied to us and we attempt to will what we cannot will to be. The body cries out through pain or other stress-related responses and often these cries are unheeded.

Human wholeness dwells in the tension between the temporal and the eternal. This is a wholeness that recognizes the spiritual as an integral part of one's being without discounting the reality of being in this world at this time.

In Western civilization the comfort of the self has been troubled for
many centuries by a bewildering polarity cultivated by those who
claim wisdom and the ability to offer us advice. We have been torn
between the gurus of science and gurus of the soul. Both have
persuaded us to believe their wisdom separately. In the experien-
tial life the division between physical and mental is not clearly
defined. We may now be on the threshold of experiencing an inner
wisdom that may heal the breach between science and the spirit.[6]

Each day I see patients who look to science for the answers to
their every symptom. There is a belief that the world of medicine
has a medication and/or surgical technique that will serve to
restore wholeness to the crippled spirit as well as the discomfort-
ing physical symptoms. When healing does not occur, the patient
tends to blame the medical practitioner, and when a cure is obtained, the practitioner is viewed as the healer. Seldom does the
patient recognize his/her own role as a partner in the healing
process. This particular view of healing has been fostered by the
medical profession and has often been a source of irritation for
both the professional and the patient. The professional is in the
position of being looked upon as a failure if the treatment does not
work, and the patient is in the position of feeling betrayed by the
gurus of science and may feel helpless and hopeless when he or
she does not get well.

What is often ignored in illness patterns is the role of the will
and how this influences not only the current health status of the
patient but the patient's ability to attain a state of wellness. A
disordered will is the result of using the will to will what cannot
be willed. If the symptoms can just be decreased, everything will
be all right, the patient thinks, but what is overlooked by the
patient is the fact that the symptoms have occurred because everything is not all right. The following cases may serve to clarify this
statement.

Sam was a 45-year-old male executive. He was referred for
chronic gastrointestinal discomfort that mainly occurred within a
half hour after eating. The patient was over six feet tall and
weighed one hundred and thirty five pounds. He had symptoms

of stress, but his intestinal discomfort was what he was most concerned about. Sam looked tense but did not want to discuss his condition. I asked him if he wanted to stay. He stated that he had sought help from his physician and was not happy about his referral for biofeedback pain therapy. He would stay, however, for at least this one session. He then shared the fact that he had a history of ulcers and colitis. In the past he had obtained relief through his medications. This was the first time that he had failed to gain a significant decrease in his pain level with medication. His physician wanted to avoid stronger measures and had referred him for biofeedback therapy.

Sam described himself as a self-made millionaire. He owned his own company and stated that he was happiest when he was working. He reported to work at 6:30, five days a week, and sometimes went to work on the weekends. During the day Sam ate light snacks at his desk and his pain was manageable. Sam's wife insisted that he take a "dinner break" around 5:30 each afternoon, and it was this meal that was, in his words, the source of his pain. He often returned to work in the evening, but his pain lasted for several hours. It was, he stated, "the major annoyance in his life." "It is bad enough to take this unnecessary break, but the pain afterwards is really annoying."

You cannot impose your own will on the patient, but rather need to meet each patient in his/her own place. Sam came from a place of successfully applying his will to attain his personal goals. He had a flourishing business, financial security, and a wife who placed very few demands upon his time. He was angry about the daily interruption for the "dinner hour," but he also realized that it was not an unreasonable request. "My wife knows that my work is my life and she places few demands upon my time. I earn the money and she spends it." Sam did not have children, and he did not have friendships outside of his work-related associations. He stated that he liked his life just the way it was, but he did not like his pain.

Sam was willing to try pain therapy, but he admitted that he did not believe that it could really help him. He had hoped that the physician would prescribe a stronger medication, and he was disappointed that pain therapy had been suggested. Sam felt threatened by this type of treatment program because it was a movement toward the will of the first realm. This made it necessary to focus on direct, practical methods of reducing his discomfort. He agreed to complete five sessions of therapy. I began by emphasizing ways to increase the effectiveness of his present medications. I pointed out that his anger and impatience, especially in relation to the dinner break, increased his stress level and made it more difficult for his medications to effectively decrease his symptoms. We worked on basic tense-relax exercises and ways to incorporate "mini-breaks" throughout the day. These were all time-efficient and Sam liked that. We worked on what he ate and how he ate his dinner meal. He became more aware of the fact that he ate too fast and did not sufficiently chew his food. In time Sam gained a sense that he could help to decrease his symptoms, and this in turn gave him a sense of control. Sam kept his agreement and completed five sessions of biofeedback therapy. He attained modest results and seemed to feel that his time had been well spent. He did not want to deal with underlying issues related to his discomfort and I had not pushed him to do so.

Walter, a 41-year-old management executive, was referred after an initial psychiatric consultation. He was given medications for symptoms of anxiety, but he had requested biofeedback therapy. He had heard about biofeedback therapy and wanted to see if he could benefit from such a program. Walter had filled out a short questionnaire, and during our first session we discussed his answers and talked about his concerns. He did not have a pain problem, but he did have chronic anxiety and reported that he often felt out of control. I asked him to tell me about his work. "I usually have at least three projects going on at any given time," he said. "I feel driven to work and when I am not working on a project I cannot relax. The funny thing is that most people do not see me as being driven. I think that I make a hard job look easy and that there is some resentment because of my success. I don't need to work at the management company because I've done well on my own projects, but I still work like it was my only job. I set the pace and those who work for me have to put their work first and their personal life second. They are paid well, the production level is high, and there is a very small turnover rate."

I said very little, as it was a time for listening. Walter spoke in a relaxed way. He looked comfortable and had a pleasant manner. He had left college after two years and joined the management firm. "I have worked for the same firm for the past twenty years, and I am now one of the top executives. I have also invested money along the way, and I could easily retire and live on my investment income. I have a lovely home, a vacation retreat, a loving wife, and a 15-year-old daughter. I have everything that I set out to have, but I feel anxious every time the work schedule slows down. I find myself looking for a new investment project as soon as one project is about finished. The only time I really relax is when we go to our vacation retreat, but after a week or so I leave the family there and go back to work. My goal is to be able to enjoy my financial security, to feel closer to my wife and daughter, and to find satisfaction in areas outside of my work."

While I am listening to a patient, I am doing just that and nothing else. It is, as mentioned earlier, a basic component of the patient–therapist dialogue. It is possible to listen while planning out treatment strategies or writing down notes, but one cannot be fully present when one is doing two things at the same time.

Walter and I met, we talked, and then we started to plan. I explained that it takes time to decrease symptoms and that while the exercises might appear to be simple ones, they could profoundly affect one's sense of well being. Thus, we started with the breath. Our breath is our life, and any time that the breathing rate is changed there is a chain reaction that has to do with the state of our being. One can become chronically stressed, and any change, even for the better, may cause symptoms of anxiety. When one has anxiety after a traumatic event, it is uncomfortable, but also understandable. If one feels anxious when one is relaxing or if anxiety awakens one from a deep sleep, the symptoms are traumatic. Many times these symptoms feel life-threatening. The whole body goes into an emergency mode. It is not unusual for a person to feel that he or she is having a heart attack. The heart is pounding, the breath is labored, the body becomes sweaty and/or clammy, and fear sets up a state of panic. This is an acute stage of anxiety, but many people do not reach this stage. They reside in a state of chronic anxiety that creates a sense of not being safe in the world. This is not a matter of logic, but rather a matter of feeling. It is the worst kind of enemy because it cannot be clearly identified, and it permeates the whole body. This is where the realm of the second will fails us. Walter had achieved wealth and control over much of his world through utilizing this aspect of the will, but he knew that he wanted something more.

I wondered what had prompted Walter to request biofeed-back therapy. He stated that his secretary had been my patient. She had been treated for migraine headaches and had significantly decreased her symptoms. I was surprised and pleased by the connection. I remembered how she had described her "boss." He was, in her words, a person with high expectations, but he was also generous and appreciative.

I asked Walter when his symptoms bothered him the most and when he felt least anxious. He stated: "I am always somewhat anxious, but I can cover it up by keeping busy. When we go away to our vacation retreat, I do well for a few days and then the anxiety starts creeping back into my life. Sometimes I am very anxious when I am completing a business transaction. I think that I am torn between a compulsion to take care of every detail and a fear of the void that will be left when every detail is completed."

Before completing this initial session of biofeedback therapy, we worked on relaxed breathing and started with a deep breath in through the nose, deep into the lungs, and then exhaling through the mouth. It was a long exhale and there was a sound of tension being released. This was not a normal breath, but rather a "signal breath" that reminded the body to slow down. This breath was the foundation for our work. In time it was coordinated with a calming image that made it a more comprehensive exercise. During each biofeedback therapy session I added additional components of the biofeedback therapy program. These components included reducing smooth- and skeletal-muscle tension, visualization, pacing skills, and a home practice program. Walter explored what it meant to let go of some of the control in his business life and to experience what I have referred to as the will of the first realm.

One day, after about fifteen sessions of biofeedback therapy, Walter stated that he had decided to take a year off of work. "I want to spend more time with my family, especially my daughter, before she is fully grown and on her own." Walter had carefully planned out what he wanted to do, and I was supportive of his plan. He wanted to travel for a month in Europe, take a class in art history, spend time at his vacation retreat, and just stay home for awhile. He felt that he would have time to enjoy special activities with his daughter and to learn to enjoy quiet times on his own. I suggested that he keep a journal, which he did.

Walter completed twenty sessions of biofeedback therapy over a period of six months. At first he was seen on a weekly basis, but after fourteen sessions there was a tapering-off period. During the biofeedback treatment sessions he had explored what it meant to let go of some of the conscious control that he tried to impose upon every aspect of his life. I encouraged quiet walks, not so much for physical exercise, but more as an exercise in being in the present. The child lives in the moment, but, in time, concerns about the future may obscure the moments of his/her life. We all live with uncertainties, but when we are busy trying to control what we may not be able to control, tension and anxiety will develop. Being in the present is a way of establishing a sense of balance between the realms of the will. It is not a matter of one realm being more desirable than another, but rather that we need both realms of the will for our health and wellbeing. Guided imagery, focused concentration during the biofeedback session, and being present myself all served to help Walter experience aspects of the will of the first realm. Here, too, were some of the components that helped to build a healing dialogue.

Walter felt confident about the year ahead and looked forward to his time off from work. We both knew that it was time to discontinue his biofeedback therapy. He was ready to work on his own and we had worked to develop resources for home practice. He was still seeing his psychiatrist, who continued to monitor his medications.

I saw Walter shortly after he had successfully completed his year off of work. He stated that he felt closer to his family and more in touch with his own needs, but admitted to some difficult times. He was taking one project at a time and he was trying to balance his work, family, and personal-time schedule. "My hardest job is to keep from running away with myself. I am trying to take some time to relax and enjoy what I have in life." He was still taking medication and utilized the biofeedback therapy techniques on a regular basis.

Walter did not return for additional biofeedback therapy, and I did not see him for almost two years. He stopped by my office to say hello, and we had a brief discussion about how he was doing. He stated that his medication had been changed and that he was "doing just fine." I was somewhat dismayed because he was so lethargic. He had gained weight and seemed to lack his natural vitality. One of his business projects had not turned out well, but he stated that he was "taking it all in stride." I wondered what had precipitated the change in Walter's medications. He mentioned a new diagnosis, but he did not indicate that there had been a time of increased anxiety. He seemed to be pleased that he was so relaxed, but I was uncomfortable because he seemed to be too relaxed. I felt a sense of loss. This was not a natural state and Walter's spirit seemed to be veiled behind the effects of his medication.

My last contact with Walter was by phone. I called to see how he was doing about six months after his visit to my office. He stated that he had continued to have business difficulties, but his voice sounded stronger and he indicated that he was fine. I wished him well and let go of my need to check on his progress. This, too, is an important step in the healing partnership.

Both of these cases point to the issues that arise when the will of the second realm takes over. The body becomes an object to be overcome. When symptoms arise, they are treated as something outside of one's being and as an enemy that must be kept under control. It is not uncommon to hear someone say that a particular part of their body is acting up or that they have to get rid of a headache or a stomachache. As the split between the mind and the body widens, the frantic efforts to silence the body become more desperate. It might appear, from the patient report, that Walter was less driven by his willfulness, but he had been silencing his body with medications for many years, and it was only when the symptoms of anxiety became severe that he sought professional help. He was, in his own words, ready to do whatever was necessary to decrease his symptoms and to feel more in balance. In the case of Sam we see a patient that still feels in control and simply wants to get rid of an annoyance in his life. He generally functions well and has very little motivation to change his lifestyle.

Anxiety and Depression

In his article "Merchandising Depression," Farber refers to the 1950s as the Age of Anxiety. This was also the period when tranquilizers became popularized through mass-marketing procedures. As Dr. Farber points out, it is sometimes necessary to classify a disorder in order to sell a product that will cure that disorder. From the Age of Anxiety we moved into the Age of Depression and again the promise of relief was as close as the corner drugstore.

> Is it any wonder that sufferers are glad to fling aside the particularity, the messy concreteness of their private torments and enlist in the ranks of Depression, where the only forced marching will be back and forth to the pharmacist?[7]

It is not that the states of anxiety and depression are in any way new phenomena but rather that we tend to view them in the abstract rather than in relation to the individual and his/her life situation. The elimination of symptoms becomes the focal point, and it is generally believed that antidepressants and tranquilizers will, depending on the type of symptoms, offer the necessary relief. When we treat people suffering from symptoms of anxiety and depression with pills, they may feel better but the person, as a whole, is not addressed. Dr. Farber points out that one must accept some responsibility for one's condition and that this is the hard and painful process that is involved in attaining a healthful state.

Many of the patients that I see are both anxious and depressed. They have become increasingly anxious over increased symptoms, and this tends to become a vicious cycle that exacerbates the symptoms and the anxiety. The patient often feels depressed because he sees himself as the victim. The body has taken over, and he is ruled by pain, anxiety, phobias, or any number of other symptoms that have increased in frequency and intensity over time. The patient feels out of control and the will to will what cannot be willed becomes a way of life. As the symptoms worsen, there is a concurrent decline in the dialogue with his symptoms of distress and between himself and the world.

The infant and young child does not try to control the body, but over time he/she is taught to control bodily functions and to withstand various discomforts that occur from injuries, illness, and/or an emotional reaction. The child tends to act out in relation to discomfort because verbal skills are limited and there is more of a general body response because the nervous system is not yet fully developed. The dialogue with one's own being and with the world are intricately bound together, and a delicate balance must be maintained in order to maintain one's health.

Once we have learned to control basic body functions, it becomes easier to ignore internal messages and to use the will to gain more control over the world of things. The early warning signs of stress can be ignored without too much distress, and involvement in the world of things helps to override the signals. The hands may be cold, failure to respond to the need for elimination may cause constipation, muscles may be tense due to inactivity, and the eyes may be suffering from improper lighting.

Still the individual keeps working, and the symptoms may be ignored for many hours before they reach a level that cannot be ignored. It is possible, over time or due to trauma, that the symptoms will worsen and that the signals of distress will become habitual and it will be impossible to ignore them. At this point the will may be used to try to will what cannot be willed. The pace may become more frantic; anger, depression, anxiety, and increased symptoms tend to surface. The uniqueness of each person is very much in evidence when it comes to health, and the patterns of illness very clearly demonstrate this fact.

Laura was a 26-year-old junior executive with a communications firm. She was the older of two daughters and had been married for one year. She had a very demanding job and twenty employees reported to her on a daily basis. The patient was referred for biofeedback because of frequent headaches. She had multiple medical problems including erythema multiform, menstrual irregularity, anxiety attacks, and various food allergies. The patient was a pleasant, attractive, young woman who did not appear to be in any acute distress. When asked, she stated that most of her symptoms began to surface during her college days. During that time she worked 30 hours a week and maintained a full college schedule. She described herself as driven, perfectionistic, calm, and anxious. She played tennis and did some jogging and liked to do well at whatever she did. During one session the patient stated that she felt obligated to do well to make up for her sister, who was much less achievement-oriented and was a disappointment to her parents.

This patient was unable to see the relationship between her symptoms and her stressful lifestyle. She had little time for recreational activities and tended to play as though they were work. By this I mean that she needed to win and would not stop or limit an activity even if she was very tired. It is not unusual for such patients to continue to add additional stresses to an already stressful lifestyle, and in this case, the patient continued to function well but developed additional symptoms. She began to have gastrointestinal discomfort, fatigue, and episodes of dizziness. Laura wanted medical help to decrease her symptoms, and for her this meant medications. She had never considered altering her lifestyle and did not recognize the symptoms as expressions of her own distress.

In the case of Laura it was necessary to help her to see the relationship between her symptoms and her lifestyle and how she could begin to establish a dialogue with her own being. This is not an easy task and sometimes increases discomfort for a period of time. The realm of the second will helps to suppress the inner dialogue, and when the voice is finally heard, it is usually an uncomfortable sensation and sometimes painful. What is important here is the fact that when this inner dialogue is shut off, it affects one's dialogue with the world and shuts out the will of the first realm. The individual has the feeling of being in control, but it is an illusion.

It often helps patients to realize that letting go of control accomplishes a great deal. One cannot attain a good night's sleep without relinquishing the will to do so. Taking the time to listen to a guided imagery tape helps to restore and replenish the systems that support life. The discomfort that one may initially feel is not a warning signal, but rather a resistance to change. Muscles that have known only tension for long periods of time will tend to resist any relaxation that goes beyond the momentary periods of fatigue-induced relaxation.

If one feels most comfortable accomplishing tasks, it is necessary to emphasize that a great deal is being accomplished when one takes the time to learn biofeedback-assisted self-regulation skills. I usually start with EMG muscle tension reduction because the patient can both see and feel the results of their efforts. In time we move to those areas that are more akin to the first realm of the will, but I can only move in that direction. A healing partnership guides, supports, and creates a way, but it is the patient's resources that determine the way.

Laura needed to accept, for herself, that she had limits. This was very difficult because she prided herself for exactly the opposite reasons. The more she accomplished in any one day the better she felt about herself. Sometimes a patient needs permission or a directive to do less. Most people in Laura's life complimented her on her accomplishments, but they also came to expect a great deal from her. This occurred in her professional life as well as her personal life.

The two realms of the will represent a delicate balance that is never fixed, but is, at all times, in flux. Laura learned to listen to her body signals: they were not her enemies. She had never learned to listen to her own voice, and in order to do this she had to set aside a time for communication. She learned to let go of some of the control in her life and to rely less on medications. We both felt that she had done well during the sessions and, most importantly, Laura felt ready to proceed on her own.

Notes

1. Leslie H. Farber, *The Ways of The Will: Essays Toward a Psychology and Psychopathology of the Will* (New York: Basic Books, 1966), p. 9.
2. Leslie H. Farber, *Lying, Despair, Jealousy, Envy, Sex, Suicide, Drugs, and the Good Life* (New York: Basic Books, 1976), p. 6.
3. Ibid., pp. 6–7.
4. Ibid., pp. 32–33.
5. Barbara Brown, *New Mind, New Body Bio-feedback: New Directions for the Mind* (New York: Harper and Row, 1974), p. 1.
6. Ibid., p. 353.
7. Leslie H. Farber, "Merchandising Depression," *Psychology Today* (April, 1979), pp. 63–64.

CHAPTER 7

Trauma

Chronic pain is pain that no longer serves as a warning signal. It is an entity in itself. This is true of other chronic conditions that do not cause physical pain, but persist longer than six months and disturb one's sense of well being. When one becomes a patient, one seeks to be healed. To be healed does not necessarily denote a cure. There are no real cures for tragedy, but there are possibilities of healing. Life is too complex to look for absolutes, but there is hope for less pain and an improved sense of well being. Sometimes symptoms lie dormant for years, and only after a trauma, or years of wear and tear, do they once again come to the surface. I am often reminded of the last paragraphs of Albert Camus' novel *The Plague:*

> And, indeed, as he listened to the cries of joy rising from the town, Rieux remembered that such joy is always imperiled. He knew what those jubilant crowds did not know but could have learned from books: that the plague bacillus never dies or disappears for good; that it can lie dormant for years and years in furniture and linen-chests; that it bides its time in bedrooms, cellars, trunks, and bookshelves; and that perhaps the day would come when, for the bane and the enlightening of men, it would rouse up its rats again and send them forth to die in a happy city.[1]

We all live on the edge, and there is no one who is immune to the possibility of prolonged pain. This includes symptoms that cause both physical and emotional pain. There are specific causal factors that are well known and can be referred to without diminishing the complexity of the problem; we are left with the mystery of healing. It is this mystery that provides the necessary ingredient for healing. If we knew all of the components of healing, hope would be limited, and so would the dimensions of healing. Again, I turn to Camus's Dr. Rieux:

> ... Dr. Rieux resolved to compile this chronicle, so that he should not be one of those who hold their peace but should bear witness in favor of those plague-stricken people; so that some memorial of injustice and outrage done them might endure; and to state quite simply what we learn in times of pestilence: that there are more things to admire in men than to despise.
>
> None the less, he knew that the tale he had to tell could not be one of a final victory. It could be only the record of what had had to be done, and what assuredly would have to be done again in the never ending fight against terror and its relentless onslaughts, despite their personal afflictions, by all who, while unable to be saints but refusing to bow down to pestilences, strive their utmost to be healers.[2]

Max

Max was a tall, lean man of 53. He had built and raced cars, trained horses, ranched, and lived life to the fullest, until he accidentally drove his jeep off of a cliff. He had tumbled down the cliff and miraculously survived despite multiple broken bones, contusions, and other serious injuries. Max spent the next year and a half recovering from his injuries. This included an inpatient program for the chronic pain that interfered with his every movement. Three years after his initial injury he continued to have daily pain, and he also had multiple symptoms of stress. He had difficulty sleeping, and felt agitated, angry, and frustrated. He entered the outpatient pain treatment program hoping to relieve his symptoms, but doubting that anyone or anything could help him. He had tried physical therapy, behavior modification, a transcutaneous neural stimulator (tens) unit, biofeedback, medications, and various other modalities to control his pain, but still it was, in his words, "a screaming monster that never gives me any rest."

During our first session together Max stated, "I want to be like I used to be. I can't do any of the things that I used to be able to do. I loved working on cars, but now I can hardly bend down to pick up a tool. I hurt so much that it is hard to think about anything else but my pain." Max had never really mourned his sense of loss of his former self. He was forever changed when he tumbled down the cliff and hit the ground below. His body would not let him forget the insults that had been perpetrated by this event. He had become that "screaming monster" that cried out in rage and cursed his fate.

One brief moment may bring about a metamorphosis that completely changes every aspect of one's existence in the world. For most of us change occurs more slowly, and we are given time to readjust our perceptions and expectations of ourself. Max and I discussed this issue and the fact that none of us can regain a former self. I cannot run, jump, and bring forth the physical resources that I once took for granted. Day by day I have changed, and in order to move on I must let go of the past. Here there is, for the most part, a reasonable balance between what has been lost and what is to be gained by letting go of the past. This process of change is not without pain and sadness, but most of us do not live with the constant pain and reminders of a former self that was dramatically altered during what seems like an unmeasurable moment of time. Max had been denied the passage of time that might have eased his losses, but we could not start with what he had been. I acknowledged his sense of loss and the tragedy of his accident, but I also addressed the fact that he could not regain his former self. We could only work together to tap his remaining resources and to discover what was possible at this time.

In his short story "The Metamorphosis," Franz Kafka presents an example of the world breaking in on the self. As Maurice

Friedman points out in his writings, Gregor Samsa has, in the beginning, a very small plot of ground to stand on, and, when he becomes a gigantic insect and is no longer able to be the family breadwinner, he has no ground at all.

The world abounds with Gregor Samsas. They live with an invisible contract. This contract dictates that one must live up to a role, and confirmation is given only when one fulfills this role. The individual walks on a tightrope without support and without a network to catch him/her if he/she falls. When one can no longer fulfill one's role, there is a loss of one's humanity. One may feel as excluded from the world as Gregor Samsa did when he became a gigantic insect.

In "The Metamorphosis" we see how Gregor's family shows some initial concern and sympathy for his condition, but how quickly they begin to exhibit anger and hostility. The family withdraws from Gregor and ignores his suffering. He soon realizes that his confirmation has been tied to his role as breadwinner. When one role in the family is changed, it puts stress on the whole family. The more rigid the role, the more stress on the family. In time the whole family structure is at risk.

Max introduced me to his wife. She was about 20 years younger than he was, and they had a 5-year-old child. From his previous marriage he had two children who were in their early twenties. Max had prided himself on his physical prowess, and he had accumulated both property and an income that afforded a comfortable standard of living. His chronic pain was interfering with his sex life and his ability to join his wife and children in some of their favorite activities. They had all participated in off-road-vehicle adventures and horse-back riding. He had spent much of his own time working on his cars and his ranch property. These activities now caused increased pain and Max had taken to watching television and spending time by himself in his workroom. "Most activities just remind me of what I can't do, and that's most everything that I used to do."

During the first days and weeks after an injury or a serious illness, family and friends tend to hover over and support the one who is incapacitated, but the limits of each family member and friend will become evident with time. This is when anger and hostility surface. Max and I discussed how supportive his family had been during the first months after his injury, and how little they now seemed to care about his problems.

During each pain therapy session we discussed both the reality of Max's situation and his own movement behavior. Was he holding his breath when he moved from one position to another? Was he bracing to protect himself from further injury? Was he chronically tensing his upper body muscles, especially the facial muscles? He had to stop concentrating on his symptoms and consciously decrease the tension that was exacerbating his pain symptoms.

The bracing patterns that the chronic-pain patient develops are meant to protect him or her from further injury, but they also serve to increase his or her pain. A patient may not realize that he or she is bracing, and any increase in his or her pain level will not be associated with those bracing patterns. In order to change what has become a habit, it is necessary to consciously introduce another pattern. The patient is called on to relax when every instinct of preservation says to tense and brace against the possibility of further injury. This is where breathing comes in. One deep breath, coordinated with upper body tension on the inhale and muscle relaxation on the exhale, serves as a reminder to relax chronic tension. The language of the body is nonverbal. The rhythm of the breath may set the stage for either relaxation or stress. Max wanted to quiet the "screaming monster that never gave him any rest." The breath was our first step toward accomplishing this goal. Every time Max held his breath, as he moved from one position to another, he was giving a signal of distress. He needed to learn to utilize the breath to help control his symptoms and to gain a sense of increased control. I asked him to take his "signal breath" from time to time throughout the day. When he moved from a sitting to a standing position, I asked him to inhale during the tension phase and exhale as he reached the relaxation phase. Most patients are unaware of the fact that they are holding their breath while completing what were once very simple movements for them. They are too focused on the movement itself to be aware of their breathing patterns. They are trying too hard to avoid increased pain.

Max was a restless, impatient man, but he was beginning to realize that his participation was necessary to the healing process. He was the one who needed to help calm the "screaming monster" and to realize that it was not his enemy. He could not fight himself and hope to win the battle with his pain. Max had utilized his will to accomplish much of what he had set out to do in life. He was, at this point, utilizing the will of the second realm to accomplish what could not be accomplished with this aspect of the will. His willfulness only served to increase his pain.

The comprehensive inpatient treatment program that had initially helped Max to function outside of the hospital environment was one of the best in the country. Many of his current problems stemmed from the fact that he had not learned to incorporate into his daily life what he had learned to do in the more structured environment. He had, instead, increasingly turned to his pain medications for relief. Pain medications are most effective for short-term pain relief and need to be carefully monitored when used for chronic-pain relief. Max's pain medications were no longer as effective as they had once been. He needed increased medication to deal with the intensity of his withdrawal symptoms as the effects of the medication wore off every three to four hours. We worked together to increase his own pain reduction resources, and his pain medication program was restructured and more carefully monitored by his physician.

Max had never viewed himself as a partner in the healing process. He was the victim and "the 'docs' ran the show." When he failed to get the help that he needed, he resorted to taking matters into his own hands. At this point Max was willing to admit that he needed help. "I've listened to the doctors and I've also been real stubborn at times. One thing I do know is that if I'd been a horse they would have shot me by now." We both knew that it was time for Max to participate more fully in his own pain management program. He had to become a full-time partner in order to break up some of his more destructive patterns and to discover better ways to manage his pain.

You cannot dictate what is "good" for a patient. You can introduce pain-reduction methods, but they must become personally meaningful to the patient for healing to occur. I introduced relaxation tapes, tense/relax exercises, breathing techniques, and all of the standard biofeedback modalities, but at each juncture of the program I relied on Max's input about what was working for him.

Max learned to listen to his "screaming monster" and to lull him to a restful state. He was not going to go away. He became a "guardian monster" and alerted Max when he ignored his more subtle symptoms or neglected his pain management home practice program.

What was Max's home management program? He had decided what he would do and what he would not do. It was important for him to be honest with himself and with me. He would use one of his home practice tapes one time per day at least five out of seven days per week. Ideally, more frequent usage was desirable, but he knew that he would not comply with a prescription for additional practice sessions. He would walk for at least 20 minutes per day at moderate pace; no bracing under normal circumstances; "signal breath" exercise off and on throughout the day; regular breaks ("pacing") during the day; take medications only as prescribed; eat regular meals with less sugar, caffeine, and alcohol intake; take time for short walks or quiet play with his young son (he had formerly engaged mainly in "roughhousing" activities); spend some time everyday on one task that he could do, possibly with a little help (this entailed looking at what repair work he could still do on his cars); and plan "mini" vacations with his wife: one-day trips, an evening away, or quiet dinners together.

Max completed 20 sessions of pain therapy. There were periods when his progress was very limited, but by the end of the treatment period Max felt that he had significantly improved his pain management skills. I had encouraged him to develop support systems within his own community. This, I felt, would help him to maintain his present level of pain management and might also serve to further decrease his daily symptoms. Hospitals seldom offer "hands-on treatment"; acupuncture and other more esoteric treatment programs were suggested. He joined a family health club that offered massage, a whirlpool, and other amenities that eased his pain. I also suggested family counseling, and Max took this suggestion under consideration. Max and his family had undergone extensive counseling during Max's initial hospitalization, but now the reality of his condition was a daily challenge that strained his family relationships. Max's role in the family had changed. He could no longer maintain his image of the indestructible male who presided over his family. He was more vulnerable, both physically and emotionally. There were many issues that put him at risk, but Max seemed to be ready to handle his problems as best he could. He was not a victim. He was in his words, "Just hanging in there, giving every day a go at it and raising a little hell from time to time."

Jessica

Four months after a minor fall Jessica began to have daily neck and shoulder pain, headaches, and multiple symptoms of stress. She suffered from sleep disturbance, anxiety, and fatigue. She consulted her physician, but a medical examination and various diagnostic tests failed to provide any significant medical data. Medications were prescribed for her anxiety and sleep disturbance. During the next three months Jessica's symptoms decreased, but she was disturbed by the fact that she now needed her medications to control her symptoms. Her physician recommended therapy.

During our first session together, Jessica and I discussed her work, home life, and present symptoms. She had few significant stressors, aside from her current health concerns, and her health history was excellent. We discussed her recreational activities and various other aspects of her life. Jessica had a responsible job, and she had always felt in control. Being dependent on medication made her feel out of control. She still had frequent headaches and neck and shoulder tension, and this, too, was stressful.

I asked Jessica when she had last taken a vacation. She stated that she had taken a vacation about seven months previously. "I love to swim and scuba dive, and I plan my vacations around these activities. I went to Hawaii and I had a fairly good time." She hesitated, and then went on. "I had a small disaster about three days after my arrival. I was walking on the sidewalk and suddenly I was airborne. The next instant I was on the pavement. My injuries did not require medical attention, but I was shaken up. The next day I had a sore shoulder, a skinned knee, and some bruises. I took it easy for a day or two, but then I was as active as ever." "I still can't figure out how I fell. I just seemed to have tripped over nothing."

Our ground is our security in the world. Jessica and I discussed how a fall is akin to losing one's ground. When our security in the world is threatened, even for an instant, it is traumatic. Recognition of this fact may prevent the more severe symptoms that arise in a post-traumatic syndrome. Jessica had dismissed her accident as a minor incident. "I didn't want to think about my fall. There were no broken bones, and I didn't want to make a big deal about a few bruises and a skinned knee."

Post-traumatic stress is commonly overlooked or discounted by both the patient and the professional. This is especially true when there are no broken bones or other signs of physical injury. The outer wounds heal, but the inner wounds continue to fester. The inner voice can be ignored for a time, but it will find a way to be heard.

The developmental stages of our early life provide us with the basic movement skills that are necessary for the exploration of our world. We develop a sense of self as we interact with our environment and our world as a whole. We develop a place in the world and have a sense of our own ground. There is a testing of limits and the excitement of new challenges. Each child explores and creates the world anew. They tumble, fall, and sometimes give up, but their ground will stay intact if there is a "safety net to soften the blow."

We are all grown-up children and we too need a "safety net," a community of support that acknowledges our pain and loss without judging our capacity for healing. When my young neighbor accidentally fell into a rose bush, he cried out in pain. His family members gently removed the thorns and tended to his wounds. He was not lectured on the dangers of not watching where he was going nor was he admonished in any other way. His sister read a story to him, and his brother shared his bubble gum with him. Soon he was back at play and well aware of the potential danger of rose bushes.

Children take pride in their physical feats, but they also need to share their pain. Sometimes a bandage, even on a very small wound, is important. Mastering a particular skill does not guarantee infallibility. We are all vulnerable, but we are most vulnerable when we lack a community of support. Post-traumatic stress is increased when feelings are denied and/or discounted. A hug, a kind word, or a helping hand may be the best medicine. Dialogue is also healing and it is too often missing in the treatment program.

Once Jessica began to understand her symptoms, she was less fearful of them. She learned that she did not need to rely on her medications for relief. I focused on teaching Jessica to reduce her shoulder and neck tension and this served to decrease her headache symptoms as well as her shoulder/neck pain. During the treatment sessions I utilized the biofeedback equipment, but it was important for Jessica to realize that she did not need the equipment to control her symptoms.

Implicit in the treatment program was the need to re-establish an image of wellness. Jessica had formerly thought of herself as a healthy person, but the last eight months had threatened this image. We used guided imagery and self-affirmations during the sessions, and a home practice program was developed. We explored past resources and activities that had been important in Jessica's life. As she began to resume a more active life, this too

enhanced her self-image. Gradually, the post-traumatic stress syndrome that had increased her symptoms began to decrease. Jessica
developed the confidence that was needed to continue to work on
her own. She was also looking forward to her next vacation. Her
destination was still undecided.

Manuel

I have seen many patients who have suffered an extreme
trauma that did not involve any visible physical injury. One such
patient was Manuel. He had worked evenings at a small con-
venience store, and he usually worked alone. One evening several
men entered the store, looked around, selected a few items, and
then approached the payment counter. Manuel rang up the sale
and, as the cash drawer opened, one of the men pulled out a gun
and pointed it at Manuel. He demanded all of the cash in the
drawer. One man took the money, one man took additional shelf
goods, and the third man, with the gun, indicated his intent to kill
Manuel. One of the men told him to forget it and said, "Let's get
out of here." The man with the gun looked at Manuel and said, "If
you call the police or identify us in any way, you are a dead man."
He then pushed Manuel into some boxes, and all three men fled
the store.

Manuel struggled to his feet, and he called both the police and
the owner of the store. The police arrived first, and they asked him
many questions about the suspects and also about the robbery
itself.

When the owner arrived, he wanted an accounting of the
money that had been taken during the robbery. He also wanted
Manuel to stay on the job until a replacement arrived. In the
meantime, the suspects were captured and Manuel was asked to
come down to the police station to identify them. Four hours after
the robbery Manuel returned home and went to bed. He was
supposed to report to his workplace the next day, but he could not

do so. He was apprehensive about his safety, and he was beginning to experience tightness in his back and neck.

I asked Manuel about his symptoms. "I have back and neck pain. I do not sleep well and when I do sleep I have nightmares. I hate to go out of my house, and I no longer go to work. I fear for my life." The police report stated that the suspects had been on a rampage that included three other robberies. Manuel felt, however, that they might find out that he had both called the police and identified the suspects.

Manuel never returned to his workplace. He had called his employer and stated that he could no longer work there. He lived with his brother and his cousin, and they were willing to help him out for awhile. Three months later he was referred for pain therapy. His symptoms had worsened, and he also feared that he would not be able to work again.

It is hard to reverse symptoms when one is concerned about meeting one's basic needs. We all have a basic need for some sense of both economic and personal security in the world. Manuel and I discussed his financial problems. He was given the necessary forms and help that he needed to apply for disability. Next, we discussed the reality of his fears. His fears were grounded in a life-threatening event, and he had faced his own mortality. Each night he dreamed his death, and it was becoming more real than his life.

We completed our initial 90-minute session. Manuel had shared his deepest concerns and an opening had been established. Healing cannot be rushed, but it can be nurtured. That was my basic goal.

When Manuel was pushed into the boxes during the robbery, he may have sustained some bruises, but there were no apparent injuries. Trauma is a very serious injury, but it is often overlooked because the symptoms may take time to surface. It was to his employer's benefit to adopt a business-as-usual attitude, and Manuel was expected to be on the job the next day. The police personnel appreciated Manuel's cooperation, but they could not be expected to provide him with the emotional support that he needed. Manuel's brother and cousin were supportive, but they could not continue to maintain the necessary financial and emotional support that Manuel needed.

In our office Manuel was initially given medical help. This involved diagnostic tests, medications, and referrals for psychotherapy and pain treatment. The office staff addressed him by his name, and they were friendly and helpful. It is difficult to establish a healing partnership if the office environment is not warm and caring.

The patient's own voice is also very important. Manuel chose to have pain therapy, but he initially rejected psychotherapy and/or group therapy. We worked together on a weekly basis, and each week we spent part of our session discussing what was working for him as well as new and/or ongoing problems. We discussed his safety, financial problems, family issues, and other factors that affected his symptoms. The session also included biofeedback therapy and home-practice instructions.

It is difficult for most patients to understand why their trauma symptoms take so long to decrease. Manuel's back pain stubbornly persisted and encroached on his every activity. I find that the example of compressed time tends to help define the problem. During a trauma there is an inordinate amount of tension over a very brief period of time. This tension may set up a pattern of holding tension that is very difficult to reverse. It is as though the muscles are "locked" into tension, and only during periods of fatigue do they give way to relaxation. The problem here is that they tend to "snap" back into tension once the period of fatigue has ended. This "snapping back" into tension is the dynamic of spasm activity and a cause of increased pain. Spasm activity may occur after a simple movement, and the patient may become increasingly more sedentary. The need for exercise is lost in the desperate attempt to avoid the spasm activity. Healthy muscles have the ability to tolerate at least a moderate amount of exercise, and they are also accepting of the need for relaxation.

Healing is most likely to occur when the information shared with the patient is couched in language that is comprehensible to the patient. It is important for the patient to know that, sometimes, there is an increase in the pain level before there is a decrease in their symptoms. The memory of trauma fades in time but is not erased. Our body is ourself, and the memory of trauma is locked into every cell. The key that unlocks this trauma is unique to each case and this is why the healing partnership is so important. Healing takes time, and there is a need for mutual involvement between the healer and the one seeking to be healed. This is an important part of the healing partnership.

One day our secretary mentioned that Manuel seemed to be much better. I was surprised by her statement. I said that I was not sure about that. I asked her what had prompted her evaluation. She stated that Manuel was more verbal and expressive. He came into the office and initiated a conversation with the staff, and he looked more relaxed. She was right; he was getting better. Sometimes the clinical viewpoint obscures what is obvious and what is important. Manuel had a ways to go, but he was definitely making some progress.

Notes

1. Albert Camus, *The Plague.* Translated by Stuart Gilbert (New York: Alfred A. Knopf, 1961), p. 278.
2. Ibid., p. 278.

CHAPTER 8

Stress + Time = Pain

Stress is cumulative and builds up over time. Stress-related illnesses have become a major health problem during this century. It is estimated that well over half of all medical complaints and many psychological problems are related to an inability to manage the stresses of daily life. Stress itself is not a new phenomenon, but the types of stress that we must cope with on a day-to-day basis in our modern technological society demand a different response pattern if effective coping is to be achieved. Humans are physiologically equipped to handle effectively acute or short-term stress problems. The fight-or-flight response that helped ancient man to survive his/her hostile environment serves to frustrate the efforts of modern man/woman because most of today's problems are not resolved by standing one's ground and fighting, or by running away from the situation.

Stress has always been a part of life, but some researchers believe that the effects of accumulated stress have become more pervasive throughout our society. The last 50 years have produced enormous social changes, and we live in a world of uncertainties. It becomes increasingly difficult to maintain the balance between our need to cope with stress and our need to renew our depleted resources.

Walter B. Cannon, the famous Harvard physiologist, devoted much of his professional life to the development of an understanding of what he terms "homeostasis," the effort of the body to maintain organic stability. Cannon determined that strong emotional feelings such as rage and fear and various acute physical states induced arousal of the sympathetic nervous system and adrenal secretion. These changes are responsible for the fight-or-flight response and cause added stress and strain on the body. When they become chronic response patterns, they may lead to illness and/or pain.

Hans Selye, M.D., who is considered the father of stress theory, states that "stress is essentially reflected by the rate of all wear and tear caused by life." In his book *The Stress of Life*, Selye states:

> The genetic evolution of life to complex human beings was the greatest adaptive adventure on earth . . . But there is another type of evolution which takes place in every person during his own lifetime from birth to death: this is adaptation to the stresses and strains of every day existence. Through the constant interplay between his mental and bodily reactions, man has it in his power to influence this second type of evolution to a considerable extent, especially if he understands its mechanism and has enough will power to act according to the dictates of human intellect.[1]

Dr. Selye clearly points out the fact that many of our common diseases are due to "errors in our adaptive response to stress, rather than to direct damage by germs, poisons, or life experience." It is now a widely accepted fact that the types of diseases that are so prevalent in our society today are stress related and that new adaptive techniques are needed in order to improve the quality of life and to prevent the needless wear and tear on our bodies that leads to early aging and premature death.

Every person living in our modern technological society is vulnerable to stress and is likely to suffer from stress-related disorders from time to time. Then too the symptoms of stress are often variable and may occur in various combinations. At one time the psyche may be more involved in the stress reaction, and feelings of anger, irritation, insecurity, and/or "burn out" are some of the disorders that may arise. It is, however, just as likely that somatic disorders will develop. These include muscle tension, fatigue, weakness, headaches, backaches, and/or colds. Many of these symptoms are accepted as undesirable side effects of a busy lifestyle or as something we have to learn to live with. This attitude is reinforced by the medical profession, which tends to dismiss as nonmedical problems stress-related complaints that are not discernible through the usual diagnostic testing instruments. However, as Barbara Brown so succinctly states:

> Stress is the thief of health, elusive, stealthy, capricious, pernicious, and devilishly deceptive and dangerous. It is everywhere, unsettling, nettling, chafing on-again-off-again with the rhythm of life ... stress is a non-linear disease whose signs and symptoms have not yet been explicitly separated from the common complaints about the rudeness of life or its traumas.[2]

Dr. Thomas Holmes, professor of psychiatry at the University of Washington, has shown that "one of the most powerful stressors known is a sudden change in one's life situation." He ranked the death of a spouse as the most stressful life-change event and divorce, marital separation, detention in jail or other institution, and death of a close family member as being very stressful. Positive changes are also stressful, and 10 out of the 15 top crises are related to a change in family structure. Both Dr. Holmes and his associate, Dr. Richard H. Rahe, have substantiated the fact that the stress scale is applicable regardless of race, culture, and age.

Drs. Holmes and Rahe point out the extreme levels of stress that occur after a life-changing event. What is not addressed, in their research, is the effects of long-term stressors that are not, in themselves, a source of major stress. Barbara Brown emphasizes how daily stressors can also affect one's health.

> Coping with kids and dogs, budgets and jobs, gardens and cars, marketing and shopping, schools and clubs, vacations and visitors, bills and repairs are the everyday sources of stress ... Coping yes. Stress over? No. Every mini-stress causes mini-tensions of the mind and body. If the mini-tensions pile up one upon the other, mind and body cannot recover and the tensions simply add. Too much

or too frequent stresses add up to a psychic toxicity that spills over the mind coping barrier to damage the body.[3]

Barbara Brown goes on to say "Whether or not daily stresses and hassles do more damage than life-change events may, in the final analysis, be a moot point. A single event can cause smaller changes that touch every aspect of existence." If one loses a mate through death or divorce, a whole range of emotions may occur, and economic and social adjustments may cause increased stress over a prolonged period of time. The roots of the problem may go back to a life-change event, but the long-term effects of the problem will surface in the day-to-day stressors of ordinary life.

Nancy

Nancy was a young married woman with a 2-year-old daughter. She had not felt well for over a year, but extensive physical examinations had failed to detect an organic cause for her symptoms. As a last resort, she had traveled, out of state, to a well-known clinic for more extensive diagnostic tests. When these tests also failed to reveal an organic disorder, she was given a referral for pain therapy. She was suffering from frequent muscle contraction headaches, episodes of dizziness, chronic neck discomfort, fatigue, upper back pain, and sleep disturbance. I asked Nancy about her daily life.

> Before I had the baby I worked full time. I took off shortly before her birth, and I tried to go back to full-time work when she was 10 weeks old. I lasted only about four months. I began to have some pain above my eyes and fatigue. The head pain worsened, over time, and I finally took a few weeks off. I felt a little better, but I still had some head pain, and I was always tired. I tried to go back to work, but after my first week back I felt totally exhausted. I work in my in-law's business and they have been very understanding. I took some additional time off, and now I work on a part-time basis.

We need the money and I try to work about 20 hours a week. My symptoms fluctuate, and I never know how I will feel from one day to the next. I am most frightened by the dizzy spells. I forget little things and sometimes I feel like my mind is going. I don't sleep well, and I worry a lot. Sometimes I worry about dying, but now I am worrying about going back home. [At this point Nancy began to cry.] I don't know how I can face my family. Everyone was so concerned about me. I was sure that they would find a brain tumor or some other serious illness. How can I tell them that nothing is wrong with me. How can I feel so sick and not be sick?

This question presented a two-fold problem. I needed to emphasize that the symptoms were real and significant, but I also needed to emphasize that Nancy was a healthy young woman. She had made arrangements to be away from home for a maximum of three weeks. The first week had been devoted to medical appointments and diagnostic testing. She had received the results of her medical tests on Monday afternoon of the second week.

During the next three days Nancy had completed a psychological test and had been seen by a staff psychologist. She had then been referred to the pain therapy program for a "crash course." The results of her psychological evaluation were in her medical chart. She did not bring up the testing or the session with the psychologist, but at one point she stated: "I guess that my problem is in my head and not in my body." We had one week left to lay the groundwork for a more balanced view of her condition.

I did not want Nancy to leave our first session thinking that her symptoms were simply products of an imaginative mind. I stated that her symptoms were real and that both the mind and the body were working together to express her suffering. I emphasized that it would be very difficult to decrease her symptoms if we failed to take this into consideration. We needed to find ways to calm both the body and the mind. It was not a matter of two separate entities, but rather the importance of the interaction between the mind and the body.

Nancy had mentioned her 2-year-old daughter during the

session, and 2-year-old behavior provides an excellent example of how cumulative stress builds up over time. I asked her to think about her daughter's behavior when she feels the need for attention. I said, "In the beginning she might take a rather subtle approach—possibly a tug at your clothing, or an attempt to take your hand. Whatever means she employs, you can be sure that she will not be satisfied until she has your full attention. If at first you fail to respond, she will move on to less subtle approaches. If, time after time, she has to work rather hard to get your attention, she may develop patterns that are, from the beginning, hard to ignore. Of course, it is also possible that she may give up. If this happens again and again, she will internalize her unmet needs, and they may fester for many years before they erupt and make themselves known. Each child develops his or her own behavior patterns, in response to his or her meetings with family and friends."

Our patterns of handling stress have evolved over time. Most of us are taught to ignore the subtle messages of our body. We must learn to live by the clock. Children learn to eat and sleep on a schedule and to delay their bathroom needs until recess, or a more convenient time. We learn to sit for long periods of time, to control our anger, and to deny our own feelings. In time, we may use whatever means we can to silence the voices of our own being.

I emphasized to Nancy that her fears about an organic disorder were reasonable ones. What had worked in her favor was the persistence of her own warning systems. She had been forced to listen to these signals before an organic disorder had developed. Yes, it was true that the system had become over-reactive, but now she had the opportunity to become an active participant in the healing process. This process would include breathing exercises, biofeedback-assisted muscle tension reduction techniques, autogenics, visual imagery, and home practice strategies. At the end of the first session we had, I felt, established a working relationship, and Nancy was less distraught about the absence of an organic disorder.

During our second session together I asked Nancy when she had last felt well and what had helped her in the past:

I felt pretty good before my daughter was born, but after her birth I never seemed to regain my strength. I didn't have any time for myself. I felt that I should be with her when I wasn't working, and between working and taking care of her I just got worse. My mother-in-law began to help me out and my husband also helped out. The more help I got the worse I seemed to get. I did have good days, but then the symptoms would return and I'd be right back where I started.

I asked Nancy about her community, friends, and recreational activities. What, I asked, did she do for fun?

I haven't had much fun lately. We have very little money left over after our bills, and I haven't felt like doing much of anything. We live in a small town that doesn't offer a lot to do anyway. My husband has lived there most of his life. My own family lives about 50 miles away. We have been married almost three years, and we are friends with some of the people that we work with. Both my husband and I work in his parent's business, but I work in the office, and he mainly works away from the office.

Nancy was 22 years old, and there were few surprises in her life. Her daily routine moved between her workplace and the responsibilities of her home and family. She seldom took time for her own enjoyment, and she had lost sight of her own needs. She felt guilty when she took time off of work unless she was ill, and she felt guilty about the time spent away from her daughter.

Many pain patients fall into a pain cycle syndrome. They are continually trying to make up for the time lost during periods of increased symptoms. This leads to another episode of debilitating pain and a sense of lost time. This syndrome is fostered by the patient's sense of guilt when he/she does not complete work tasks when he/she is able to do so. The pain cycle syndrome is self-defeating, but it is usually very difficult to convince the patient that this is so. In order to break the cycle of pain the patient must learn to reinforce his/her periods of reduced symptoms. It is very difficult, if not impossible, to break the pain cycle until the patient begins to understand the futility of this cycle and begins to believe that he or she can reverse it. Then too there is the problem of guilt.

Few patients believe that they deserve to take time for themselves, when they have decreased symptoms. The patient may never believe that he/she deserves to take care of himself/herself, but the practical side of breaking the pain cycle may initiate a positive response.

The practical side of pain management is to increase the length of time between the patient's cycle of increased symptoms. The emphasis shifts from taking care of oneself to gaining time. There will be increasingly longer periods of time to complete tasks if one learns to "pace" himself/herself between the episodes of increased pain. The desire to do a week's work in a couple of days is confronted. The patient is encouraged to utilize the periods of decreased symptoms for home practice reinforcement exercises, relaxed recreational activities, and moderate tasks. In time the patient begins to see that he or she can manage the symptoms and increase productivity if the tension levels are decreased over time.

Nancy's symptoms were decreasing, but she was not completely happy about her improved state. She did not like the idea of her improvement being coupled with her being away from her home and family. She found it difficult to tell her husband that she was doing well, but she was also fearful that the symptoms would return as soon as she was back at home. I explained that symptoms often decrease when there is a change in one's environment, but it does not denote that one's own environment is the cause of the symptoms. Change tends to "shake up" the pain cycle pattern, and in Nancy's case it provided some time away from her usual responsibilities. She was staying with a favorite cousin, and this had provided a very supportive atmosphere. Then too, she had been assured that she did not have a life-threatening illness. While she was initially dismayed by this news, she was also healthy enough to appreciate the fact that her symptoms were benign. I had only a few more sessions with Nancy and I decided to focus on ways to help her to incorporate into her everyday life what she was learning in the pain treatment program. I returned to an earlier question. What, I asked, had helped her in the past? "I used to be more active before my daughter was born. I exercised and my husband and I used to go camping. Whenever we had a chance we would go someplace where we could hike and/or swim. Our outings decreased after our daughter's birth. I was not feeling well and it was harder to plan ahead. I never knew how I'd be feeling and it was easier to stay at home. I feel better right now and I know that it has helped me to be with my cousin. We have laughed a lot and there hasn't been any housework, grocery shopping, or other responsibilities."

My basic plan for Nancy was to introduce a new pain management concept during each session. Before doing this, however, we would discuss ways to incorporate into her daily life what she had already learned. Nancy lived in a small desert community, and I was unable to provide referral sources that would serve to reinforce what we had covered during the pain management program. The one available resource was the local recreation center. Mother/toddler classes and exercise programs were available. During the summer they offered community swimming and a variety of other programs. The fees were low, and there were times when babysitting was available.

Nancy loved her daughter, but she had not learned to enjoy relaxed times with her. She was very concerned about being a good mother, wife, and daughter-in-law. She needed permission to take time for herself, and time for relaxing activities with her daughter and/or husband. I reminded her that it was important for her to learn to play again. I suggested that she allow her daughter to be her guide. Each child has the gift of play and offers it to the adult world. From the child we learn the meaning of being present and of living in the moment. Children are natural teachers; they teach by example. I also encouraged Nancy to take some time each day for herself. Many young mothers utilize a child's nap time for household chores. I suggested that she take at least a half hour of that time for her home practice tapes or some other relaxing activity. We explored ways to facilitate family outings and ways to meet some of her needs for private time away from her family responsibilities. She decided to ease back into her work schedule and to work up to her former 20-hour work week. Both Nancy and her husband worked and socialized with her husband's family members. Nancy lived in a small community, but I expressed the hope that she would meet other young mothers at the recreation center. Many of her husband's female family members were older, more experienced women, and she needed at least one or two young women that understood and shared her own concerns. Nancy had compared herself to her very competent mother-in-law and to other female relatives who seemed to accomplish their household tasks and family responsibilities with ease. They often offered advice, but seldom offered the emotional support that she needed.

Once Nancy was back in her home situation I wanted her to feel that she had adequate resources that were readily available to her. I did not want to impose a structure on her but rather to present options. This would enable her to stay in touch with her own sense of well-being and to take some responsibility for her own health. We had covered ways to decrease her muscle tension levels, breathing exercises, peripheral warming techniques (autogenics), guided imagery, and the need for an exercise program. There would be times when a hot bath would serve to decrease her symptoms and other times when she might feel the need to listen to her guided imagery tapes. I encouraged relaxed walks and play time with her daughter and/or husband. I had confidence in Nancy's ability to utilize what she had learned in the pain management program, and I expressed this confidence to her. I emphasized that she was a healthy young woman and that she deserved to feel better. Before leaving the program Nancy and I agreed on two follow-up telephone calls to see how she was doing. I would call her in one month, and we would arrange for a second call at that time. We also agreed that a call to her husband would be helpful. It was important for him to understand and support her needs. The call was made and Nancy returned home.

I called Nancy, as promised, one month after she had left the treatment program. I asked her how she was doing. "I am doing pretty well. My husband's family says that I am more relaxed. I don't think that I have changed that much, but it is easier for me to take some time for myself. I am trying to take better care of myself."

I had never confronted Nancy about the fact that her pain problems had provided a "way out" for her. She already had enough guilt. What she needed were ways to express her own voice. This entailed both an awareness and an acknowledgment of her own needs. This is a lifelong journey, but Nancy had taken the first steps.

The second time that I spoke to Nancy she was continuing to do well. She had occasional symptoms, but they were less intense and she stated that she could handle them. She had found her own community resources and was participating in a child-care co-op and a yoga class. Nancy was continuing to work for her in-laws, but she was also doing some office work in her home. She was enjoying the flexibility of working, at least part of the time, at home. I was surprised and pleased by her initiative. Sometimes I think that I know the answers, but patients teach me otherwise. When patients begin to find their own voices, they are likely to find their own answers. This is part of the healing partnership. The healing partnership can be facilitated but the art of healing comes from a wisdom that does not consciously set out to accomplish a particular goal. It takes wisdom to know how to facilitate healing. Ben Weininger, a psychoanalyst and friend, had a way of offering simple advice that was filled with wisdom. He did not try to provide answers, but he did provide a sense of freedom that gave the other permission to seek his or her own answers. I especially like his advice to "learn, live, love, laugh, and let go." That is exactly what Ben did, and that is the legacy that he left behind.

Hans Selye ends his classic book *The Stress of Life* on a philosophic note:

> You do not have to be a professional scientist to experience the

great melodious creations of Nature, any more than you have to be a composer to enjoy music. The most harmonious and mysterious creations are those of Nature: and to my mind it is the highest cultural aim of the professional scientist to interpret them so that others may share in their enjoyment.

As children we all had what it takes to enjoy wonderful and mysterious things. When a child points out something unusual which he has never seen before—a colorful butterfly, an elephant, or a sea shell—just watch his eyes as he cries out with enthusiasm . . .

We all had this priceless talent for pure enjoyment when we were young, but as time goes by, most of us—not all—lose this gift. We lose it because, gradually, we have seen most of the things that we are likely to encounter in everyday life, and custom stales variety. The petty routine of daily problems also tends to blunt our sensitivity to the detached enjoyment of greatness and wonder . . .

. . . very few people in the usual walks of life retain the ability really to enjoy themselves: that wonderful gift that we all possessed as children. But it hurts to be conscious of this defect, so adults dope themselves with more work (or other things) to divert attention from their loss . . .

The inspired painter, poet, composer, astronomer, or biologist never grows up in this respect: he does not tend to get the feeling of aimlessly drifting, no matter how poor or old he may be. He retains the childlike ability to enjoy the impractical by-products of his activity. Pleasures are always impractical, they can lead us to no reward. They are the reward.[4]

I think that many children are natural philosophers. This is certainly true of my young neighbor, Malik. He often walks around the yard and inspects the plant life and takes note of the bugs and butterflies. He has a favorite spot by the side of the house that is full of cacti, geraniums, onion plants, and weeds. Now and then he says to me: "I love this wild area. I hope that you will leave it this way. It is nice to have a place where the weeds can grow." I think that we all need a "wild place" of our own. A place that leaves space for surprises and unexpected joy.

Notes

1. Hans Selye, *The Stress of Life* (New York, McGraw-Hill, 1978), p. vii.
2. Barbara Brown, *Between Health and Illness: New Notions on Stress and the Nature of Well Being* (Boston: Houghton Mifflin, 1984), p. 49.
3. Ibid., pp. 49–50.
4. Hans Selye, Stress of Life, pp. 443–445.

CHAPTER 9

The Silent Cry

Some disorders are potentially life-threatening, but remain silent during the early stages of incubation. For months, and sometimes years, the warning signals are absent or too subtle to discern and the disorder may remain undetected. Without accompanying warning signals even the hint of a potentially dangerous condition may be totally ignored and its very existence denied.

Among the leading causes of premature death are cardiovascular disease and cancer. "Long after other major diseases had been conquered, heart disease still appeared to come like a thief in the night. It seemed to victimize people, to snuff out their lives prematurely and without warning."[1] What appears to be a thief in the night may actually be a long-forgotten part of the self that lies in a hidden, wounded, silent state. Traumas and/or long-term stressors release irritants that serve to weaken the protective mechanisms of the individual's emotional and physical defense systems. The silence is broken and a cry of protest may burst forth with an uncontrollable venomous rage. Our predisposition for cancer, heart disease, and other disabling conditions have their roots in the beginnings of life. In his book *The Causes and Prevention of Cancer* Frederick Levenson addressed this issue.

> When the baby feels irritated, the mother soothes him, and the irritation goes from his involuntary nervous system to her. Baby's

cells continue dividing rapidly in a normal, healthy way. But if the mother periodically adds powerfully to the baby's irritation or does nothing to siphon it off, the dynamics for cancer, both biologically and psychologically, will be established. Rather than be overwhelmed and have cells die from irritation, or succumb to marasmus, the irritation is channeled into the baby's very core to be stored as a translocated gene ready to be activated in the face of additional subsequent irritation.[2]

A lack of early dialogue will affect one's whole life. Patterns of illness are developed in relation to other people and reflect the society in which we live. Psychosomatic disorders and catastrophic diseases do not just happen. We give birth to them when our emotional and physical pain is silenced. James Lynch states

> Again and again we have stressed the need for additional prospective and retrospective medical studies that begin in childhood. But we must also remember another aspect of the connection between health and companionship. Everyone's life is unique. No two people experience precisely the same social support, either in childhood or in adult life. Thus, while overall health trends can be assessed by examining mortality statistics in large populations, eventually that macroscope view must be complemented by an examination of the unique social experience of the individual. In order to bridge this gap and examine how human relationships affect the health status of individual people, another approach must be used—clinical rather than statistical—focusing on individual cases rather than large groups—an approach that follows the individual through his unique life experiences.[3]

The lack of early dialogue, compounded by subsequent losses, grief, the lack of a loving partnership, and the transient nature of our society all contribute to a breakdown in the body's own defense system. There is a turning in on the self. The body chemistry that once helped to defuse the effects of stress and pain now serves to exacerbate the symptoms. The individual is victimized by his or her own internal chemistry. Physical and chemical irritants coming from the outside—caused by, e.g., air pollution, X rays, Agent Orange, and cigarette smoke—are external (exogenous) carcinogens. The chemicals arising from within the body that cause irritation to the cells are internal (endogenous) carcinogens. These are potentially far more damaging. They are produced by the body's own defensive structure, and their immediate purpose, in limited dosage and duration, is to ward off irritation. But if the reaction is too strong or prolonged, they cause irritation. Levenson states

> Many children grow up with "carcinogenic communication." They learn the negative skills of hyperirritation and self-containment.
>
> The most carcinogenic statement that can be made to a child is, "Keep crying, and I'll give you something to cry about." This is the epitome of adding irritation to an already irritated human being ... If the child cannot expect love and soothing from his parents at these times, whom can he expect it from?[4]

Children are taught self-containment when they are isolated for showing emotion. If they are left to "cry it out" or sent out of the room until they settle down, they learn to internalize their stress. What is important here is a repeated pattern of "carcinogenic communication."

> Parent's threats can certainly cause the overt symptoms of an upset to be buried—just think how far! It is this kind of induced hyperirritation that must be avoided. The parent's rage must be controlled or the child will have internal scars from it for life.[5]

The build-up of self-produced internal carcinogens will eventually result in stress, pain, illness, and, possibly, premature death. How this irritation is manifested, however, will be influenced by heredity, early conditioning, accidents and other injuries, and the influence of outside carcinogens. Individual resources are continually tested by the bombardment of both internal and external carcinogens.

The majority of the patients that I see are desperately trying to manage their accumulated stress and pain before it manages them. Cigarettes, alcohol, overeating, drugs, excessive medication, emotional detachment, and other self-destructive patterns of behavior all serve to provide temporary relief for a self turned in on itself. Eventually the infusion of stress on stress makes it impossible to contain the rage, fear, and cries for help that may have been long silenced. If an organic disorder has surfaced it will be treated medically, but all too often the accompanying distress will be muted with a pharmacological approach. This is, at best, a temporary solution. Chronic symptoms need to be treated as separate, but interrelated, entities. This is necessary whether they are organically or nonorganically based.

Cancer cells and ulcers can be surgically removed. High blood pressure, headaches, and other nonorganic conditions may be controlled with medications, but you can not alleviate the underlying causes of these and other chronic disorders through surgery or medication. The healing partnership allows the other's voice to surface and acknowledges the other's uniqueness. Healing is possible even when the patient cannot be cured.

The following case illustrates how one can literally eat away at one's own body, and how ineffective surgery alone may be.

Joseph

When I first met Joseph, I was struck by his healthy appearance and his quiet, poised demeanor. When asked about his symptoms, he spoke in a calm, detached manner. "I am having a hard time concentrating. I have to read things a second time if I want to retain the material. I would like to have some tapes that would help me to concentrate." I addressed this issue, and I did provide some appropriate home practice tapes. On his intake form Joseph had mentioned that he had abdominal pain. I asked him about this. "I had abdominal surgery for bleeding ulcers three years ago. For two years I did not have any symptoms, but during the past year I have had some off-and-on pain. I am scheduled for some tests in about two weeks." During this first session I listened, and I introduced breathing and tense-relax exercises for home practice. What Joseph had shared with me was important, but what he had not said was possibly even more important.

Joseph was 25 years old, and he was currently on a disability leave from his workplace. He had been married for five years and he had three sons, ages four, three, and one. He lived with his in-laws in their home, and he stated that it was a good arrangement. Joseph did not complain about anything or anyone, except himself. During the second session he stated that he was often impatient and short-tempered with his children. I asked him about his own childhood. "I was not raised in the United States. In my culture boys are raised to be men. We are either friends or enemies with other men. If we are enemies we fight. If we are friends we stick together. Children were treated harshly if they disobeyed adult men, but I do not want to be harsh with my children." I asked Joseph if he allowed his children to cry. He hesitated: "I do not like to see my eldest son cry." I asked what he did when his son cried. "I tell him to stop being a baby." I asked him what had happened when he had cried as a child. "I seldom cried. Children who cried, especially the boys, were hit with sticks. I seldom hit my own children, but I am impatient." I shared a personal story with Joseph.

I had just returned from my grandson's fifth birthday party. He had invited his 7-year-old brother and five of his best friends to the party. All of his friends were 5- and 6-year-old boys. During the two-hour party there were small tragedies, and almost every boy shed a few tears at one time or another. Each child's tears had been met with a measure of comfort and concern. A lost prize was found, a skinned elbow was bandaged, a spilled drink replaced, and a guest, reluctant to leave, comforted. We discussed the fact that year by year these same children would learn to hold back their tears. Society would serve to shape their responses to disappointment and adversity.

Joseph was well aware of the disappointments and adversities in the "outside world." He had a high-stress job as a company foreman, and he was continually wedged between the demands of management and the dissatisfactions of the employees. He had to produce results despite delays in materials, poor quality control, a shortage of trained employees, and the unreasonable demands of corporate management. Joseph could not vent his frustration and rage against this "outside world" and he did not want to take it out on his family. He took it out on himself. Joseph did not cry or otherwise show emotion. He bled internally and he was often in pain.

I wanted to give Joseph permission to be playful with his children. I have mentioned before that children can help to heal their parent, but that it is not their responsibility to do so. In meeting his children, and participating in their world, he could face some of his own inner scars. There was a mutual need between father and sons that provided an opportunity for healing and growth.

During our second session together I encouraged Joseph to set aside some uninterrupted time for his home practice sessions. I also encouraged him to plan some quiet sharing time with his wife. He needed to set limits on his time by planning special periods of time for himself and for his family members. During each pain therapy session I introduced at least one pain management concept. I utilized the biofeedback equipment, provided home practice tapes, discussed pacing, visual imagery techniques, and the need for exercise and focused relaxation exercises. Joseph was doing well and he had the added support of a newly initiated psychotherapy program.

Joseph continued to have periods of abdominal discomfort and medical tests were ordered. The results of his diagnostic tests showed scar-tissue damage from his first surgery and more bleeding ulcers. His physician had recommended surgery as soon as possible. I asked Joseph how he felt about the impending surgery. "I think that it will help me, and I am just waiting to hear about the surgery date." Joseph did not show up for his next scheduled appointment.

Ten weeks after Joseph's last appointment I stepped out of my office and I saw a gaunt, young man filling out some forms. It was Joseph. He stated that he had suffered a setback after his surgery, due to internal hemorrhaging. He was now recovering, but he was still weak. During the surgery over half of his stomach had been removed and the scar tissue removed. Joseph stated that every time he left the house his sons wept. "They think that I am going back to the hospital. I told them that today I was going to a place that was going to help me to stay out of the hospital. I assured them that I would be back for dinner." Joseph filled out his papers and scheduled his next pain therapy and psychotherapy sessions.

Some people are treated medically for years, and they do not get better. They are patched up like an old inner tube, and it is not surprising that yet another damaged area soon surfaces. Eventually, the whole structure is weakened and the patient is usually labeled as chronically ill. Seldom are the causal agents addressed and the long-silenced patient may feel hopeless.

Sometimes I say to a patient that we need a period of just standing back to see where we are. We need to take time to dream and to face our fears. It takes courage to change, but only then can we exit from our own bondage. Every change necessitates some loss and this too must be acknowledged.

Bob

Bob's health problems had forced him to take an early retirement. During the past eight years he had suffered two heart attacks and a multiple by-pass operation to repair his damaged heart. He had a 20-year history of high blood pressure and various stress-related disorders. Bob was over 55 years old, and he had been referred for therapy because of frequent chest-wall pain and constant stress-related back and shoulder pain. He was under the care of an internist and a cardiologist, and each had prescribed certain medications, which he continued to take on a daily basis.

I looked at Bob's intake questionnaire. It was the most detailed and beautifully executed intake form that I had ever seen. I mentioned this to Bob, and he stated that he had been in a line of work that demanded accurate, detailed reports. "It is just a matter of course for me to be as thorough as possible at whatever I do."

During this first session we discussed Bob's symptoms, his lifestyle, the treatment program, and what he hoped to gain from the program. "I want to get rid of this chest pain and other depression- and stress-related symptoms. I feel like I'm constantly on the verge of another heart attack." I asked him what he was now doing to help himself. "I take my prescribed walk every day, keep track of my blood-pressure readings, and only do light work around the house. My wife works and I am enjoying doing some of the cooking." I gave Bob a home practice relaxation tape, and I asked him to set aside an uninterrupted time for twice-daily practice with the tape. One week later Bob called me from the hospital. He had been hospitalized due to increased chest pain and a possible heart attack. "My cardiologist asked me if I had been doing any additional work or exercises. I told him that I had been doing a relaxation tape that included some upper-body tense-relax exercises. He told me that I should not have been doing this type of exercise." I told him that I would send him another tape, and that I would call him in one week. I sent Bob a tape that did not have any movement exercises in it. One week later I called again and we scheduled a second session of pain therapy. He was recuperating at home and seemed to be doing well. Both Bob's intake form and his experience with the tape helped me to plan a more effective treatment program for him. His intensity and drive for perfection lacked the discrimination that was necessary to sort out what was worthy, and what was not worthy, of his intense effort to measure up to his own self-imposed standards.

During our second session Bob discussed what he presently considered the greatest stressor in his life—his father-in-law. The

"Colonel" was over 80 years old, and he had been living with Bob and his wife for the past few years. During much of Bob's married life the "Colonel" and his now-deceased wife had lived close-by, but after his wife's death he felt it was the duty of his only daughter to take him into her home.

Now that Bob had retired, he wanted some time for himself. His father-in-law expected Bob to help him during the day, and to make matters worse, he continually insisted upon having his own way. "For years the 'Colonel' has presided over every family affair, and his ready wit has placed him center-stage. He is also critical and demanding, but around the kids he is usually entertaining, and they love his jokes and stories."

Bob wanted his father-in-law to move into a nearby retirement hotel. His wife agreed that her father should move out of the house, but each time the subject was brought up, he refused to discuss it. I asked Bob if he realized that his father-in-law's presence in the house was detrimental to his health. "You have worked hard for the past 30 years and you deserve to enjoy your retirement, and to protect your health." I gave Bob permission to do what he knew needed to be done. What surprised me was the speed with which it was accomplished. The "Colonel" was moved into the retirement hotel within a month. He soon had a whole new audience for his stories and jokes, and Bob had regained his home.

We were now free to address other issues that contributed to Bob's symptoms. We worked on developing pacing skills, and on giving only a minimal effort to less important tasks. Bob was an accomplished artist and an aspiring poet. I encouraged him to devote more time to those activities that expressed his creativity. He also loved fishing and had always dreamed of owning his own boat.

For about three months Bob's symptoms decreased and he appeared to be doing well. Then, he began to feel increasingly fatigued. Medical tests were ordered and the possibility of either bleeding ulcers or colon cancer was discussed. The tests were all negative and further indications of internal bleeding were negative. Bob's color and energy returned and he talked about getting the fishing boat that he had always wanted. His family contributed money to the project, and Bob soon had his boat. He had wanted that boat for years, but somehow the money had always been needed for household bills or other family expenses.

Bob had discovered his own voice. For years he had put his needs aside for the sake of others. There was a sadness when he spoke, but there was also a sense of completion. He had returned to his art and he had also realized his dream of navigating his own boat. His chest pain was still present, and it served to warn him when he neglected to pace himself.

Bob's family loved him and when he began to express his needs and concerns, his family listened. They were supportive and encouraged him to take care of himself. He is not cured. Bob still does too much, too well, but he is better. He has slowed down and he takes breaks. Most of all, he is enjoying being at home without his father-in-law.

When I last saw Bob, I told him that I liked to think of him out on his boat, free from the constraints of time; I see him exploring and enjoying the openness of the sea. He smiled and seemed confident that he could now get along on his own.

After deciding to include Bob's story in this chapter, I asked him if he would consider illustrating his pain artistically. Here are two poems that he wrote: one when he was depressed and in pain, and one when his symptoms had decreased.

Depression and the Pelican

I had a dream the other night
that I'll not soon forget
about a frightened pelican
trapped in a piece of net.

The more he fought to free himself
the more tangled he became

but when we tried to cut him free
he thought we were to blame.

He turned on us with all his rage
so we had to let him be.
He struggled toward the pounding surf
and plunged into the sea.

The tangled net weighed far too much
and he sank beneath the sea
I woke with a start as I realized
that Pelican was me.

I am caught in my own heart's net
will someone cut me free,
Or must I like the pelican
find peace beneath the sea.

—Bob Sprosty

On Wings of Faith

We stand before the restless sea
like shifting grains of sand
and dream of what our lives might be
if we would take command

From a simple grain of sand
a pearl born in an oyster shell
may adorn a jeweled crown
Yet rising in the endless sea
our dreams are tumbled down

Take heart, dream on!
For man is not a captive thing
bound firmly to the shore;
with faith, he'll climb on frigates wing
to freely rise and soar!

—Bob Sprosty

Notes

1. James J. Lynch, *The Broken Heart: The Medical Consequences of Loneliness* (New York: Basic Books, 1979), p. 18.
2. Frederick B. Levenson, *The Causes and Prevention of Cancer* (New York: Stein and Day Publishers, 1985), pp. 46–47.
3. James J. Lynch, *Broken Heart*, p. 86.
4. Frederick B. Levenson, *Causes and Prevention of Cancer*, pp. 127–128.
5. Ibid., p. 128.

CHAPTER 10

Creating an Image of Well Being

Our image of well being is always in flux. Every cell in our body is in constant communication with other cells, and the complex systems made up by these cells are responsive to the conscious and unconscious communication of our mind. The language of cells is sensory and precedes verbal communication. There is a life-sustaining rhythm that must be maintained, and even subtle changes in one's psychological and/or physiological state may be interpreted as a threat to the whole organism. This is especially true when the threat is associated with pain. When pain or any other condition becomes chronic, the constant message of alarm strains the whole of one's being. The pain may be limited to one area, but the effects will be global.

To decrease symptoms and reverse established patterns, a new message needs to be introduced and incorporated into one's whole being. There are multiple pathways, but the mind is the main communicator.

Panic attacks provide an excellent example of the power of the mind and the extreme state of distress that results when the mind and body are united in an emergency response. The term "panic attack" has come to mean a condition that occurs when danger is not imminent, yet the panic attack has the same effect that a life-threatening event would have. Under normal circumstances a state of panic is directly related to an event. It is a stimulus–response behavior that is caused by extreme fear. When a panic attack occurs without an identifiable stimulus, the attack itself becomes the stimulus, and a chronic state of fear reigns within the whole organism.

When treating a patient suffering from panic attacks, it is important first to acknowledge his or her condition. Occurring, as they do, without obvious provocation, panic attacks send out a message that one is in a life-threatening physical state. The person's image of well being is shattered at that moment. Recovery from a panic attack does not dispel a person's fear of the symptoms and one begins to live in the shadow of the unpredictability of the attack.

Lynn

Lynn was 36 years old when she had her first panic attack. She was relaxing on the couch, watching a favorite television program. Her children were sleeping, and her husband was on his way home from a late night at the office. She was tired, but otherwise did not feel bad. I asked her to tell me about this initial panic attack.

> I was just sitting there on the couch and the next thing I knew my heart was pounding against my chest. It was racing so fast that I could hardly get my breath. I felt like I was going to die. I thought I was having a heart attack. I was not aware of time, but it felt like it went on for a long time. Later, I realized that it had not lasted very long, but afterwards I was so tired that I didn't try to move.
>
> When my husband arrived I began to cry. He wanted to take me to the emergency room, but by this time I was better. I just wanted to go to bed, but I promised to make an appointment for a check-up the next morning.

Lynn's physician had given her some routine tests and prescribed some medication. She assured Lynn that she was healthy but told her to call if the symptoms persisted. I asked Lynn about her work and her home life.

Friends and family members are always telling me that I do too much, but I like to stay on top of things. My husband and I both work hard, but we have a nice home, two great kids, and enough money to keep up with the bills. It is very important to me to keep my house clean, spend time with my daughters, and to do well on my job. My husband sometimes tells me to take it easy, but if I do that then the work piles up. As it is, I spend most of my weekend catching up and preparing for the next week. I have very little time for myself, but I am not complaining.

The medication had helped to decrease Lynn's symptoms, but she had continued to have an underlying feeling of anxiety. This had gone on for about a month, but then she was awakened in the middle of the night by a second panic attack. She was unable to go to work the next day, and she again consulted her physician.

Lynn's physician ruled out an organic disorder and did not want to prescribe stronger medications. She suggested that Lynn see a psychologist and/or a biofeedback pain therapist. At first Lynn resisted the implication that she had anything other than a medical problem, but she needed help so she followed up on the referral. The psychologist arranged for group therapy, and helped Lynn make the necessary arrangements for a consultation with me. Three months had passed since her first panic attack, and she was now averaging one attack per week. One had occurred while she was a passenger in the car, and now she was concerned about driving.

I explained to Lynn that ordinarily a state of panic is an emergency response that relates to survival. In her case, the emergency response was a false alarm, and it was serving to undermine her sense of well being. There may have been many subtle warning signs that had been ignored along the way, but now was not the time to address this issue.

The breath is the first line of defense. Our breath is our life, and it can work for or against us. The holding of one's breath or an unexpected quickening of the respiration rate may produce an alarm response. A slow, deep breath can be used to decrease tension and to impart a sense of calmness. Much can be accomplished with this calming breath. Shallow breathing produces poor oxygen exchange and more tension in the upper chest and shoulder area. Deep breathing brings in more oxygen and utilizes the capacity of the lungs. There is a momentary pause and then a slow, deliberate exhalation through the mouth: Inhalation through the nose, exhalation through the mouth. The patient is learning the rhythm of tense-relax and one important way to consciously influence that rhythm. During the slow exhalation phase the mouth is slightly open and the jaw is relaxed. This facial relaxation exercise is eventually expanded to include the upper body. The breath is coordinated with increased upper-body tension during inhalation and a release of tension during the slow exhalation phase. This short period of increased tension facilitates the release of excess muscle tension. This is not a normal breath, but it is, in Charles Stroebel's words, a "quieting response." The language of the body is utilized, and the message is one of calming. It needs to be repeated off and on throughout the day, and eventually one's awareness of increased tension is coupled with a response that serves to prevent a state of chronic tension.

I wanted Lynn to leave our first session feeling that it was possible to reduce her current symptoms. I emphasized that daily practice was important, and I gave her a home practice tape. I knew that it would be difficult for her to practice on a daily basis with her tape, but she would be able to utilize her breathing exercise throughout the day. The combination of focused relaxation and physical exercise was much needed, but it would take time for Lynn to make her own needs a priority.

Patients with chronic pain and/or chronic symptoms face the task of learning to meet the symptoms without being consumed by them. This takes a state of calmness and detachment that can only be attained when the patient's level of fear has been decreased.

Every time Lynn began to feel her heart quicken, she was paralyzed with fear. It was a natural reaction, but like chronic pain, panic attacks are seldom life-threatening, and fear only exacerbates the symptoms. We had to work on learning to respond to her symptoms in what seemed, on the surface, an unnatural manner. She would visualize herself as being relaxed and unafraid of her panic attacks. When she felt the first hint of a panic attack coming on, she needed to utilize her breath to abort or at least decrease her symptoms. Some patients with chronic pain breathe into the area but remain detached from the pain. To utilize these self-relaxation strategies one must practice them during symptom-free periods.

Lynn had two young children and we discussed how often, throughout the years, she had calmed their fears. Now she needed to be the mother to herself. She had grown up learning to nurture others, but she had become accustomed to letting her own needs go unmet. We talked about those areas of her life that could be modified to allow more time for herself. She presented a great deal of resistance, but I reminded her that she had already accomplished a great deal by making a commitment to her group therapy and pain treatment sessions.

Many young women need permission to accept nurturing for themselves. Like Lynn, they try to be perfect mothers, perfect housekeepers, loving family members, and perfect wives. If life is not perfect, they may blame themselves. Lynn seldom denied any request. She sometimes worked overtime to cover for other employees, baked cookies for school functions, helped coach her daughter's soccer team, hosted the family potluck dinners, and ministered to the needs of everyone else in the family. She was the first to help out at a dinner party, and the last to leave the clean-up committee. She was luckier than many women in that she had a husband to share both the financial and emotional needs of family life, but she tended to feel guilty if she did not do what she felt was her share of the work. This appeared to be most of the work, but Lynn could not, at this time, imagine doing less. I focused on trying to help her to say no to any new requests. Here we met with some success.

We began to address some of Lynn's earlier warning signs of increased stress. She had for some time been having sleep disturbance and at least one headache per week. She also had difficulty relaxing. She had reached a point when she only "let down" when she was too tired to do anything else. She had been able to ignore her earlier symptoms, but the panic attack caused a crisis that could not be ignored. We began to work on creating some time for her to meet some of her own needs. Lynn began to see that her panic attacks were not, as they initially seemed to be, unrelated to the whole of her life. We moved between practical everyday suggestions that related to Lynn's lifestyle and the development of images that restored her sense of well being.

During each session with Lynn I utilized the biofeedback equipment, and there was a period of time set aside to coordinate her self-regulation skills with guided imagery practice. Sometimes this was her only period of practice, but she did begin to have decreased symptoms. She began to demonstrate an ability to decrease the muscle tension levels over the face, neck, shoulders, and upper-back areas. Lynn became more aware of her own needs by recognizing the subtle inner messages that were continually communicating the state of her being.

One does not change another person, but you can help them to accomplish their own goals for change. Lynn did not like having panic attacks, and she wanted them to stop. As she began to see that she could gain some control over the panic attacks, she was motivated to continue to help herself. A conscious image of well being emerged from Lynn's sense of increased control over her symptoms. The message of well being was, however, first communicated by the calming messages that resonated throughout her body as she re-established a physiological and psychological rhythm that represented an image of well being. This sense of calming gave a deeper meaning to what it was that she was doing. Her respiration rate decreased, her blood pressure decreased, her skeletal muscles relaxed, her hands and feet warmed, and her brain waves shifted from the dominant, beta, thinking mode to the more relaxed mode of alpha. Lynn learned to visualize scenes that promoted well being, and she began to feel refreshed after practice sessions.

Lynn was beginning to realize that she was too grown-up and too responsible. She needed to play now and then and to express her own needs. This did not come easily, but we searched for inroads to facilitate this process. She was learning to take mini-breaks during the day, and this was both helpful and time-efficient. She would take her quieting breath and give herself a calming affirmation. She had a favorite visual image, and she incorporated this into her mini-breaks. She walked on the weekends, but was not willing to do more exercise at this time. I took my cues from Lynn; I did not try to force my own goals on her. I was pleased when she shared her perspectives with me, and there were times when I knew that she was making progress.

> The other day I took my shoes off and waded into the ocean. I ran away from an incoming wave, but I didn't quite make it. I enjoyed myself, and I didn't worry about the sand in the car. I didn't pack a lunch, and we picked up something at a fast-food place. It was fun, and I actually relaxed. I still have my moments, but I'm a lot better. There is hope for me.

She laughed and I knew that she was right.

I believe that the muscle spasms that often contribute to chronic-pain problems have something in common with the symptoms that trigger a panic attack. Muscle spasms and panic attacks usually occur without an identifiable trigger, but there is an identifiable pattern. It consists of a repeated cycle of tension–fatigue–spasm or panic attack–recovery. Muscles that are held in a state of sustained tension over long periods of time begin to lose their ability to accept the natural flow from tension to relaxation and back to tension. The muscles do not relax, but they do become fatigued. When the fatigue phase eases up, the muscles "snap" back into tension. Such episodes are commonly referred to as muscle spasms, and these spasms are a source of much pain. The tense-relax cycle is interrupted, and there is an accumulation of stress. When there is sustained tension over a long period of time or an extreme amount of tension over a short time, the tension is often vented on the self. It is at this point that one begins to consciously lose one's sense of well being, but the process may have been going on for years.

A healthy muscle accepts both tension and relaxation and moves easily between these two modes. Most people with chronic pain tend to become increasingly sedentary, and this causes increased muscle weakness. The ability of the muscles to tolerate a reasonable workload diminishes. A cycle of chronic pain and disability becomes incorporated into one's being, and eventually the chronic-pain patient sees himself/herself as living in constant pain.

Like chronic pain, panic attacks do not just materialize out of nothing. Their roots are embedded within the body long before one becomes aware of the increased tension that is setting the stage for a panic attack or some other stress-related condition. One's "inner voice" is silenced and the facade of control is maintained. Eventually, tension gives way to fatigue, and sleeplessness, irritability, nightmares, shakiness, and one or more other stress-related symptoms may eventually surface. When one has a panic attack, there is a dramatic acceleration in the process, and the loss of one's sense of well being is keenly felt. There is a loss of control, and the person lives in fear of another attack. This is very disturbing to other family members because the person has usually presented a strong image of control and others have relied on this person's strength.

The strength of the muscles and of the psyche depend upon a balance between tension and relaxation. When one is out of balance, there is an overload on one or more systems, and in time this overload will be communicated to the whole of the organism. The effects may be life threatening, or they may serve to warn against further damage. To restore health is to establish a balance that facilitates healing. It is here that the healing partnership may come into being.

Don

Don was a physically fit 26-year-old man with an excellent health history, but his sense of well being was in jeopardy because of his fear of becoming HIV-infected. As far as he knew none of his previous sexual contacts had been HIV-infected, and currently he was being careful not to put himself at risk. All of Don's diagnostic tests had indicated that he was not HIV-infected, but this had not relieved his fears. He knew that the virus could remain dormant for as long as five years, and this was one source of his anxiety. Don had also witnessed the devastation and suffering that occur when one is dying from the effects of the disease. Colds, a chronic cough, night sweats, and other related symptoms all served to increase his anxiety and his fears of being HIV-infected.

It is important for each person to realize that his/her body systems are initially orchestrated to promote wellness. Individual resources vary, but the potential for healing can be enhanced. We need to teach survival skills that focus on strengthening one's own innate capacity to repair and restore one's inner environment. Too often the focus has been directed toward conquering and eliminating a known or unknown adversary. This attitude has been fostered by alarmist media reports and the medical profession. The patient is too often viewed as a victim, and his or her own resources are diminished by feelings of helplessness and hopelessness. One cannot afford to become a victim if one wants to maximize one's own resources for healing. One needs to establish supportive partnerships that focus on healing.

Charles Garfield, in his writings, emphasizes the psychosocial elements of survival. Many of these elements might well serve most effectively if they were implemented before the onset of a life-threatening illness. Garfield asks the following questions:

How do human relationships reduce stress and affect the course and recovery from illness? What factors in a supportive relationship help induce health? Can the quality of a person's relationships significantly improve his or her chances of overcoming life-threatening illness? Although research on these issues is scarce, many people believe that caring, supportive relationships can appreciably increase the will to live and positively alter a patient's chances of survival.[1]

Garfield's writings on survival relate to the coping strategies of Holocaust survivors. He states, "Important analogies exist concerning the nature of life in extremity and psychosocial elements of survival." He goes on to ask, "What can we as helpers do to mobilize best the psychosocial elements of survival?" From Garfield's article, I have selected some of the important elements that enhance survival and give meaning to life. Garfield credits Terrence Des Pres, the author of *The Survivor*, for the following observations on survival.

> The survivor is aware of the drift toward indifference and the moment when a simple expression of care pulls him together.
>
> Some minimal fabric of care, some margin of giving and receiving, is essential to life in extremity.
>
> Survival is a collective act.
>
> Every morning a survivor's will has to be renewed: not through some secret fortitude of the heart, but through the physical act of getting up.
>
> Survivors acquire a capacity for adapting, and make the most of each day's opportunity for getting through that day. Survivors not only wake, but reawake, fall low and begin to die, and turn back to life.
>
> The need to help is as basic as the need for help. Through compassion we close the distance between one condition and another. As long as the division between unearned luck and unearned disaster remains a structure of our common world, compassion has about it the nature of a moral imperative, but only for those whom fate has not tried.

Garfield notes that Des Pres's observations show the strong relationship between the emotional state of a person and his/her physical status. Garfield states:

In time we will learn more about the psychosomatic conditions that enhance survival. We will understand better the psychophysiologic variables that promote health and even the kinds of human relationships that emotionally and physically enhance life the most.[2]

A sense of well being cannot exist alongside a victim pose. One needs survival skills to cope with the challenges of everyday life, but a challenge to one's well being calls forth all of the individual's resources for survival. Don's fears of HIV infection set in motion a possible threat to his existence. He needed to develop survival skills that would help him to conserve and strengthen his own resources for healing.

After several sessions of learning basic calming exercises, we began to focus on the development of a healing image. Don's fears had been quieted, but we needed to do more than this initial first step. His messages of fear were entrenched both in his conscious and unconscious mind, and a new message of wellness needed to be formulated. He had access to the conscious mind, and it was here that we began our efforts to establish a renewed sense of well being.

The first images to emerge were ones of nature. Waterfalls, ocean waves, quiet pools of water, streams, meadows, tropical islands, and lush green forests were all sources of peaceful images, but Don's favorite image was a hilltop that overlooked a beautiful valley. We utilized visual-imagery tapes, guided-imagery tapes, self-guided exercises, and music. Don found several of the music tapes most helpful. Eventually, he found a way to introduce the healing effects of his visual image to his whole body. He created a sacred healing place, and during his imagery practice he would spend a part of his time in that very special place. Warm vapors would spread throughout his body, and they would calm his fears and promote healing.

Once Don recognized his own healing resources, he gained a sense of freedom and personal power. This crucial step helped to create an improved sense of well being. He was ready to work on his own, but he also had a strong community of support, and this too promotes healing.

Notes

1. Charles A. Garfield, ed., *Stress and Survival: The Emotional Realities of Life-Threatening Illness* (St. Louis: C.V. Mosby, 1979).
2. Ibid., pp. 3–6.

Belief
A Triad of Healing

Every person is, in some way, a living testimony to the possibility of healing. I would find it difficult to treat a patient if I did not believe that healing could take place. This does not mean that there is necessarily a measurable change, but it does mean that the wholeness of the individual is addressed and enhanced.

Belief can be defined as confidence, faith, and/or trust. These factors are also important in the healing partnership. The triad of the patient, the therapist, and what occurs between them is vital to the healing process. This is called nonspecific healing and it is sometimes referred to as the "placebo effect." The conventional allopathic medical model relies on specific measurable results that are referred to as scientific evidence of healing. Whatever one's frame of reference may be, belief will have some effect upon the outcome. This fact brings forth the importance of the "placebo" effect. Herbert Benson states:

> When we dissected the placebo effect a number of years ago, we found three basic components: One, the belief and expectation of the patient; two, the belief and expectation of the physician; and three, the interaction between the physician and the patient . . . It appears from a number of avenues of research that when the pla-

cebo effect, or belief is coupled with the relaxation response, the patient is able to bring forth health-promoting changes.[1]

Only recently has the scientific community taken a serious interest in the placebo effect. The area of study called psycho-neuroimmunology has reunited the mind and body in relation to health and illness. Genetic, environmental, and individual behavioral factors are being more fully investigated. The effects of love, belief, and the patient-therapist relationship are less often addressed and have yet to be fully embraced by the scientific community. They are more often the unacknowledged factors in the healing arts that remain cloaked beneath medical jargon that makes sterile the very life of the treatment program.

In his article "Belief and the Management of Chronic Pain," David Bakan states that the deliberate use of belief for therapeutic purposes may lead to deceit, trickery, and misrepresentation of truth. He equates this fraud with certain placebo therapies. In his article, "The Faith That Heals," Jerome Frank questions the use of the term placebo effect, but goes on to elaborate on its basic tenets.

> This is not the time or place to review the many examples of the healing power of expectant faith, usually referred to by the unfortunate term "placebo effect," that is, the response of patients to inert medications. The strength of the placebo effect depends on a complex interaction between the momentary state of the patient, the physician, and the current environmental setting, but on the average it is far from trivial.[2]

It is unfortunate that within the medical community the placebo effect has been compromised and trivialized by the manipulation of the patient's beliefs to obtain desired research data. What is important in the placebo effect is the accumulated scientific evidence that belief affects the mental state of the patient and that the patient's mental state affects bodily processes that affect one's health and illness patterns.

> The patient, suffering from life-threatening symptoms approaches the treatment with a mixture of apprehension and hope that ren-

ders him especially susceptible to psychological influences. His expectant faith is enhanced by the surgeon's explanation of the procedure, which is based on a belief system both share, and which is reinforced by elaborate preparatory examinations utilizing impressive scientific gadgetry. This builds up to the climax, a dramatic, expensive and impressive operation in which the surgeon stops the patient's heart, repairs it and starts it up again. The surgeon literally kills the patient and then resurrects him. Few faith healers can make an equally impressive demonstration of healing power.[3]

Belief in Western medical technology creates a mental state that is conducive to healing. However, when this particular medical model is presented as the only alternative, many people are left without hope. The medical community has tended to exclude all but its own kind, and this has limited the scope of their treatment programs. This is especially true for the multitude of people that suffer from chronic pain. Meditation, biofeedback, and numerous other treatment modalities have the potential for greatly enhancing the more conventional Western medical treatment programs by helping to create an improved mental/physical state. It has been shown that almost any modality that one believes in has the potential for healing, and conversely even the most sophisticated medical treatment may fail if belief in the treatment program is lacking.

Conventional medicine has encouraged belief in the capacity of the physician to orchestrate healing through his/her knowledge of the human body and the use of sophisticated technology. This, as Goldblatt points out, is treatment that is based on a vertical relationship.

The patient assumes the inferior position of abject ignorance and faith in the physician. The doctor is viewed as holding a superior position of knowledge and power. Only with this vertical differential in position can the doctor be seen as the insurer of good results. This kind of vertical relationship is a traditional, paternalistic view of doctor and patient, but with one twist: the elements of trust and an understanding of the inherent fallibility of medicine are missing. Instead of a beneficent, learned but fallible knower the physician is viewed as a technological guarantor. . . . Doctors and patients became less friends and more independent contractors, strangers with a temporary connection.

In a vertical relationship the patient is less likely to appreciate his/her own capacity to facilitate healing and a healing partnership seldom comes into being. An alternative to this type of relationship is one that emphasizes shared decision-making. Goldblatt suggests that medical doctors need to develop "greater sensitivity concerning their responsibilities toward both their profession and their patients." She goes on to say

We need to re-educate ourselves. We are presently too demanding and too lazy. We want quick fixes for problems that often require self-control rather than medication.[4]

Andrew Weil has studied therapeutic systems throughout the world and has identified their common factors. He states that every system fails some of the time and that their success ratios cannot be fully explained by the theory or methods that support the treatment. He comes to the conclusion "that belief alone can elicit medical cures."

Belief in a system of treatment varies from practitioner to practitioner and patient to patient. Such variations can explain why any system works some times and not others. Since belief alone can elicit healing, the occasional success of treatments based on absurd theories is not mysterious. . . . Given the importance of belief as the crucial factor determining the outcome of treatment, it is necessary to look closely at the interactions. By understanding the indirect relationship between treatment and healing, people will be able to take more responsibility for their own bodies and be better prepared to make intelligent choices of treatments and practitioners when they decide to seek outside help.[5]

Weil reintroduces the question of the placebo effect or, as he refers to it, the placebo response. He comes to the conclusion that it is likely "that any favorable outcome of any medical treatment may be due, at least in part, to a placebo response." The placebo response is seen as a threat to "scientists who are dogmatically attached to the materialistic model." What makes the placebo response even more complex is the effect of nonverbal communication. The belief in the physician is viewed as vital to therapeutic outcomes, but this belief must also penetrate the patient's deeper, possibly unconscious, levels of the mind. The placebo response involves the natural ability of the body to heal when a healing environment exists. Weil states

> The best treatments are those with safe and valuable intrinsic effects that focus the belief of both doctor and patient and so function well as active placebos, unblocking innate healing by a mind-mediated mechanism while also working directly on the body. This is psychosomatic medicine at its best and good medicine by any standard of judgment, not quackery or deception. In fact, the true art of medicine is the ability of a practitioner to select and present to individual patients those treatments most likely to elicit healing from within.[6]

Weil's writings emphasize the triads of belief, the healing partnership, and the basic components of healing.

> I recognize three dimensions of belief in placebo responses to active treatments: the patient's belief in the method, the doctor's belief in the method, and the patient's and the doctor's belief in each other. If all of these factors work optimally, even procedures based on ridiculous theories can produce real cures. If they do not interact productively, even the most scientific and rational treatments may fail to cure.[7]

The three components of healing are reaction, regeneration, and adaptation. In terms of chronic pain and/or chronic symptoms there must first be a response to the symptoms. When pain is associated with a trauma the person may not be able to respond fully to the event for months or even years. Denial, self-medication, or other means of masking the pain or discomfort prevent healing. Regeneration within the body is, in some cases, limited, but the potential for regeneration of a more optimal physical/mental state is not fully known. Learning to adapt is often a matter of confronting the limits of one's own resources and the availability of outside resources. There is a reality factor that must be dealt with, but too often it is not reality, but rather the fear of failure or unreasonable demands that block effective adaptation. We are, throughout our lifetimes, going through the process of reaction, regeneration, and adaptation. When the elements of the healing partnership are combined with this process the quality of life is greatly enhanced.

In presenting Jenny's case, we have the opportunity to give recognition to the unpredictable "unknowns." It is the "unknowns" that contribute to the mystery of healing. They also remind us that identifying, categorizing, predicting, and all other scientific endeavors cannot rule out the possibility of the particular: the unique individual response to a given situation.

Jenny

Jenny was a 20-year survivor of terminal cancer. She was now 60 years old and fearful of her current symptoms. She believed that her cancer had returned. She had undergone extensive diagnostic testing, the results of which had all been negative, but it had not relieved her fears. I asked her to tell me about her cancer illness.

> When I was 40 years old I was operated on for ovarian cancer. After the operation was over the doctor told me that he had done what he could, but that the cancer had spread and he could do no more for me. He said to get my life in order because I had a year, at the most, to live.

I asked Jenny how she had responded to this news.

> I was sure that he was right. My mother, sister, and an aunt had all died of cancer, before the age of 45. I felt that I would be the next to go.

But Jenny had not died and I asked her what she felt had happened to change the course of her disease.

> Well, I'm not sure, but I do know that my decision to take a trip was a good one. I quit my job, sold many of my belongings, rented my house, and jumped in my car and headed for the Northwest. I didn't have a timetable and I felt totally free. Every day was a new adventure. Along the way I saw a few friends and relatives, but mostly I just enjoyed the scenery and took time to explore each new place. I didn't think about my cancer, because I was feeling good and I didn't have any symptoms. After about six months I decided to head back home. I wanted to clear up some loose ends and I also wanted to die at home. Well, I went home and I made an appointment to see my doctor. He seemed surprised that I was still feeling well. He examined me and ordered some laboratory tests, which all came back negative for cancer. So here I am, twenty years later. He, by the way, died five years ago, so I managed to outlive him.

I asked Jenny about her current symptoms and what, if anything, had recently been a source of stress for her.

> My greatest stress was the death of my niece last year. She was only 37 years old and went so quickly. She had the family plague, ovarian cancer. It wasn't just her death but also her suffering that really bothered me. She had been so pretty and lively and toward the end it was hard to believe that the person dying was actually my niece. I have had this pain (she pointed to her upper groin area) for some time now and I feel like the "grim reaper" is finally catching up with me. I am afraid of the pain.

During the next few sessions we worked on relaxed breathing, warming techniques, and other self-regulation strategies. Jenny began to see that she could reduce her pain symptoms. I believed in her capacity for healing, and she was beginning to believe in herself.

We discussed the fact that we must all die and that none of us know for sure how, when, and where this will happen. To become self-absorbed in our fears is to give them a reality that they would not otherwise have. Sometimes we dream our death and sometimes tragedy or near-tragedies bring us face to face with the possibility of death, but most of the time we live our lives as though we are permanent fixtures in what we know is a finite world. Jenny had done very well for 20 years and we discussed what had given her strength along the way. I asked her what had helped her to feel more relaxed. She enjoyed walking and she had enjoyed gardening before her move to a smaller apartment that did not have a garden area. I encouraged her to do some indoor gardening. We discussed how important it was to nurture not only herself, but something outside of herself.

Jenny completed six sessions of pain therapy over a period of eight weeks. She had a significant reduction in her pain level after the first two weeks and the additional sessions were utilized to reinforce her initial improvement. It was important for Jenny to realize that she did not need me or the biofeedback equipment to maintain her improvement. She had demonstrated that she knew how to reduce her muscle-tension levels, and she was able to achieve a state of relaxation by focusing on her image of a peaceful garden.

"I close my eyes, take several deep breaths, and then walk through my own imaginary garden. The more I practice the better I become at both imagery and relaxation. I like the thought that I have a beautiful garden that dwells inside of me." Jenny was also creating some beautiful dish gardens in her kitchen. One day she brought me a cactus dish garden, and I knew that it was her farewell gift for me. When I think of Jenny I am reminded that we can never know, in advance, what is possible for any given patient. What we do know is that it is possible to defy the odds.

There are patients who defy the odds, and their own determination and will to live cannot be discounted. That too is an important part of the belief component; belief that the seemingly impossible is possible. However, we cannot equate death with failure. How can anyone know the resources of another when we cannot know the limits of our own resources? Throughout life we need the support of those who believe in us, but this is especially true when we are faced with a life-threatening illness or chronic pain. This support strengthens our own resources.

Nathan

Nathan believed in himself, his patients, and the conventional medical procedures that he successfully used to facilitate patient healing. He was a healer, an artist, a loving family member, and a respected member of his community. Nathan exercised, watched his diet, and generally took good care of his health. He was also a perfectionist, and was used to being in charge. He practiced medicine in a way that has previously been referred to as a vertical patient/physician relationship. He was warm and caring, but he also felt that he was in a position to know what was best for his patients. Nathan had given very little thought to alternative medical practices because he had obtained excellent results using conventional methods and he believed in the science and technology of conventional medical science.

Over a two-year period Nathan had suffered a death in his immediate family, a failed business investment, and additional family stress. He had a history of ulcers and he began to have some symptoms that indicated the possibility of recurring ulcers. Nathan checked out his symptoms and had a series of diagnostic tests. All of the tests were negative for ulcers or any other organic disorder. During the next year the symptoms persisted and worsened. At this point Nathan sought a second opinion. This time more extensive tests were ordered and the results were devastating. He was suffering from an especially virulent type of cancer that had somehow managed to be overlooked during the earlier examinations and diagnostic testing. He felt betrayed and desperate. He knew that early detection of cancer was important and that precious time had been taken away from him. Now he was in need and he sought out the best that medical science had to offer him.

Each specialist Nathan saw explained the deadliness of his disease. It is questionable whether any of Nathan's physicians believed that he could survive the steady spread of his cancer. They shared their concerns and the fact that the odds were against him. He had little opportunity to be the patient because he was also viewed as a colleague. He needed to be a patient and at times he cried out against the technical explanations that he was forced to endure. Before each medical intervention he was given a full explanation of the procedure and all of the possible side-effects and dangers inherent in the treatment. He traveled great distances to find a cure, and he underwent various experimental operations that promised only a sliver of hope. Nathan was injected with poisons, and he was treated surgically at least six times, but each time the cancerous growth within him proved to be mightier than the forces from without. Nathan had never explored his own resources for healing, but he was encouraged to do so by a desperate family member.

I was asked if I would be willing to see Nathan and to help him to develop some visual imagery techniques related to healing. This type of invitation is difficult to accept and difficult to turn down. I knew Nathan, but I was unaware of his illness. We met from time to time at one social event or another, and he had always seemed to be in good health and very much engaged in his work and family life. I admired and respected him, and I enjoyed the spirit of love that was so much a part of his family life. I felt that it would be an honor to work with Nathan, but I also felt the responsibility that comes from agreeing to provide help when one is close to being a last resort.

The first time that I saw Nathan he was recovering from one of his many surgeries. He looked thin and tired, but he also retained some of his usual vitality. We talked about his illness, his operations, his fears, and what it was that I hoped to accomplish with him. He needed to feel in control and this was an important aspect of our working relationship. I guided him through breathing exercises and a pattern of healing affirmations. Nathan was receptive and at one point he smiled and said, "I know what you're doing—you are introducing me to self-hypnosis."

For several months I saw Nathan on a weekly basis. During each session we worked on some aspect of self-regulation and I guided him toward the development of his own healing image.

We explored images of his past and present that gave him a feeling of relaxation and peacefulness. We were making progress, but as Nathan's presurgical strength returned so did his resistance. During the time that I worked with him, I began to see a pattern emerge. After a surgical or chemical intervention Nathan would be open to imagery work, but as his strength returned, he would put up barriers and would state that he knew what to do. In each case his returning strength seemed to be interpreted as a signal that the latest medical intervention had eradicated his disease. He would return to work and our sessions were often cancelled during that time. Nathan's conscious mind denied his illness, but whether the messages of his physicians and/or his own inner voice could be silenced was another matter.

During one session Nathan shared a dream that we both knew had to do with death. Nathan was in a tunnel and he was being drawn toward a bright light. He felt that he could feel the touch of the loved one who had died and that it was warm and comforting. This dream occurred during one of Nathan's post-surgical recovery periods, and it was a stronger image than any of his healing images had been. I attempted, on this occasion as well as other occasions, to encourage Nathan to seek out other types of support. He was unwilling to see anyone but me and his own physicians, who were only available when he was having a pre- or postsurgical problem or a significant change in his symptoms.

I continued to see Nathan until I had to leave the country for an extended period of time and during that period Nathan died. Nathan's passion for life is his legacy. He wanted to live and he had a family that never stopped its own battle to save his life, but the forces of life and death are always in a delicate balance. We have limited control over our unconscious mind, and the hurts and fears that sometimes emerge from this part of our mind communicate with our cells in a language that has great impact on the life of the cells. The shattering of one's belief system; the constant assault of surgery and/or chemical compounds; the lack of belief in one's own healing ability; the loneliness of pain, fear, and anger;

the loss of a loved one; and the limits of one's own resources all come into play. Despite this, one cause will be singled out. Cancer was the end result, but it was not the whole of the problem.

There is a difference between wanting to believe and belief. Nathan believed in statistics, surgery, physicians, and pharmacology. The statistics told him that there were few, if any, long-term survivors of his disease. This was especially true when the disease had progressed for as long as his had before being treated.

Every physician that he sought out was willing to operate on him, but they were also brutally honest about his chances for a complete recovery. They, too, believed in statistics. Each recurrence of his disease further eroded his belief that a cure was possible.

Nathan's own resources for healing were diminished as he faced one failed surgery after another. Every part of his body reverberated with his anger and his fear of death. During the day his conscious mind kept him distanced from his feelings, but at night and at other vulnerable times it was not life but death that stalked his whole being.

Did science fail Nathan? Not completely. He had gained time, and time is precious. Without surgery and pharmacology Nathan might have died much sooner but he did not receive what he believed he deserved. He had given many people the gift of hope and this he did not receive.

You cannot share the intimacy of another person's pain and struggle for life without feeling the impact of that pain. Nathan shared his dreams, both of life and of death. I saw the ebb and flow of his life energy and I heard him cry out against the onslaught of his disease. Sometimes dread and anger would consume him, but more often he would be focusing on the future and his concerns about his family and his work. His intellect, his sense of humor, his artistic abilities, and his love of life were never dimmed for long, until death silenced all that he had been.

It is important for me to recognize my own limitations. I mourned the death of Nathan and I cannot discount the limits of my own resources. Life energy is tapped when I work with dying patients, and I live with the impact and void that their deaths create. I also live with the memory of a remarkable human being, and I am thankful for that gift.

In returning to belief, it is important to recognize that it is a "gut-level belief" that changes the course of disease. Andrew Weil states

> It is based on experience as well as thought and must be psychosomatic to begin with, bridging the barrier between modern cortex and primitive brain stem. . . .

Weil sees this necessity as a cause for both hope and despair.

> It means people cannot just will themselves to be healthy or set their innate healing mechanisms in motion whenever needed. It also means they are likely to be conscious of the ways they now block healing, stress their bodies, and create susceptibility to external agents of disease by sending negative mental energies through those same mechanisms. . . .

There is power in belief and the mind is able to modify the body in ways that promote healing. "This should make people much more aware of their own potentials to deal with illness and adversity. . . ."

> It should also motivate both doctors and patients to find better, safer methods of allowing healing to occur, such as the use of active drugs that evoke placebo responses but cause fewer adverse reactions . . . Research on new psychosomatic therapies has already produced techniques such as biofeedback and systems of relaxation and visualization that really change physiological problems for the better.[8]

Weil feels that research on mind/body communications will be "the frontier of medicine in the twenty-first century." If this is true then there is hope for both a flourishing of preventive medicine and a lessening of human suffering.

Notes

1. Herbert Benson, "Looking beyond the relaxation response: An interview with Herbert Benson," *Revision*, Vol. 7, No. 1 (Spring 1984), p. 51.
2. Jerome D. Frank, "The faith that heals," *Johns Hopkins Medical Journal*, Vol. 137, (1975), pp. 128–131.
3. Ibid., p. 130.
4. Ann Dudley Goldblatt, "Warning symptoms," *The University of Chicago Magazine* (Fall, 1989), pp. 14–20.
5. Andrew Weil, *Health and Healing: Understanding Conventional and Alternative Medicine* (Boston: Houghton Mifflin, 1983), p. 195.
6. Ibid., p. 218.
7. Ibid., p. 227.
8. Ibid., pp. 253–254.

CHAPTER 12

The Gift of Hope

When I think of medical treatment I usually think of examinations, diagnostic tests, pharmacology, and surgery, in that order. Symptoms are identified and treated, but the patient may not be addressed beyond his/her symptoms. Norman Cousins states:

> Physicians will give no guarantee that medical treatment will "cure" any given case. Neither will anyone who ministers to the emotional or spiritual needs of a patient provide absolute assurances. But human beings are energized by their hopes. A patient's will to live cannot be totally disregarded in making a prognosis or in drawing up a treatment strategy. It is necessary to mobilize all the resources of the patient—physical, emotional, intellectual and spiritual.[1]

To mobilize the patient's own resources does not offer false hope. It offers the support and guidance that is needed if one is to test the limits of one's own resources. Hope does not thrive in a climate that does not foster the patient's own capacity for healing. I have never agreed with the policy of giving patients a "death sentence." We all know that life is a finite condition, but hope comes from the knowledge that all of the factors that sustain life cannot be fully known. I have personally encountered numerous individuals that were told, by their physician, that they had anywhere from three months to a year to live. This is a very powerful message from a very powerful messenger. I think that physicians can deal honestly with their patients without becoming messengers of death. They must, however, recognize that their own limitations need not determine the criteria for the patient's own capacity for healing.

What I have said about patients with a life-threatening disease is also true for the patient who suffers from chronic pain or other chronic symptoms. These patients are often given a "life sentence" and it may be similar to the one that was given to one of my patients. "We have done everything that we can do for you. There is a limit to what medications can accomplish and surgery is not an option. I know that it is not easy to learn to live with this pain, but I have nothing further to offer you." This particular patient did not give up. She requested a pain therapy program and she learned that it was possible to decrease her symptoms. Luckily, she had done some reading on her own, and she had learned that other options did exist. There is a need to move beyond doing something to the patient and to help the patient to help himself/herself within the healing partnership. When this happens there is hope, and an image of wellness is possible.

Our friend Hayim died twice and lived two lives. I did not know him during his first lifetime, but I did meet him during his remarkable second life. Few of us experience being face to face with our own death, but most, if not all of us, can identify with one or more life-changing events. How we respond to change is related to our sense of hope. Many people, in their response to life and death, give us the gift of hope. Others, by helping to sustain and nurture us, give us the resources to maintain hope. Hayim, during his second life, showed us what hope can accomplish.

Sherman, as he was known during his first 47 years, had been, in his own words, a "hard-hitting" businessman. "I drank a lot, ate a lot, worked a lot and yelled a lot." Sherman worked in the entertainment business. He knew many people, but he had few friends and/or close relationships. He had been divorced once, widowed once, and he had been a "mostly absentee father" to his daughter. He was, in his words, a workaholic and he measured his life by his success at work and the money in his pocket.

The last day of Sherman's first life was much like any other day. He had worked sixteen hours, and he was preparing to leave a party that had been, like most parties that he attended, more business than pleasure. He remembered feeling a sharp pain in his chest, but he had no memory of what had happened next. By the time the paramedics had arrived his heart had stopped beating. They were able to resuscitate him, but his heart stopped several times on the way to the hospital. Modern technology and a skilled medical staff brought Sherman back to life, but the prognosis was not good. He remained, for some time, on a life-support system.

What Sherman remembered about his time in the hospital and his year-long inpatient/outpatient treatment program was the care that he received. He often stated that the staff had given him hope. At first he had wondered what was so great about being alive. He would never work again, and unless he changed his whole lifestyle he was facing imminent death. The staff helped Sherman to see that he had the ability to make whatever time he had left meaningful and fulfilling.

Sherman had dropped out of college in his twenties to pursue his career in the entertainment industry. Now he wanted to go back to college to complete his undergraduate degree. He not only did this, but went on to graduate school. Sherman began to work with my husband, Maurice Friedman, who was his mentor, and he studied Religious Studies and Humanistic Psychology. He immersed himself in his studies and his student life. He lived simply and very frugally. I met Sherman during this time and found him to be brusque but likable. He liked to say whatever he wanted to say in the fewest words possible, and he was not one in general to express personal feelings. He did express his desire to establish a Center of Hope for the dying and others who were faced with a life-threatening illness. Sherman felt that this would be his way of expressing his gratitude for the hope that he had been given during his own life-threatening illness.

Sherman had never been a religious man, but he had a desire to learn more about Judaism and his Jewish heritage. He developed an independent studies program and moved to Israel to continue his course work at the Hebrew University in Jerusalem. My husband continued to serve as his adviser and helped him to meet his academic requirements. Sherman immersed himself in his studies and was soon very much at home in Israel.

In 1987, my husband was selected to be a Senior Fulbright Scholar at the Hebrew University. It was during our time in Jerusalem that I began to know and appreciate Hayim, as he now called himself. We would walk through the university hallways and students of all ages would greet him. He was well liked and respected by the other students and the professors. He continued to live a Spartan lifestyle, but I never heard him complain about his health or his living conditions.

Hayim completed his booklet on *Hope* while we were in Jerusalem, but his dream of a Hope Center was still being formulated. He wanted the booklet to be given out, free of charge, to dying patients and their families. It was a work of love and of thankfulness to those whom had given him hope in a time of despair.

During our time in Jerusalem I was aware of Hayim's health problems, but I was also aware of how beautifully he managed his pain and limitations. He was thin and pale from the chronic oxygen insufficiency that sometimes slowed him down. Yet he managed to traverse the difficult stair-strewn path up to our home in Jerusalem and to cover the distances between his classes at the university. He had learned to pace himself and to accept his condition in a way that did not limit his enthusiasm and full participation in his various activities. Hayim's chronic chest pain had become his companion. It warned him and it tempered his activities, but it did not rule his life. He was a free man and he made the most of his opportunity to be just that.

Hayim was sad to see us leave Israel and we were sad about leaving. But our work was in the United States. We said our good-byes and left for home. The next time that we spoke to Hayim was by telephone. He had called to tell us that he was dying of cancer. He had lived for 13 years knowing that his heart might give out at any time, but he had never expected to die of cancer. This was a blow that crushed his own hope, and it was difficult for him to talk to us. He died a short time later. Hayim left very little in the way of material possessions, but he did leave us all his legacy of hope in the form of the booklet which he prepared for his center.[2]

HOPE:
MY RESPONSE TO DYING

In the beginning
came divine contractions,
it was the Creator
at work making room
from within Himself
for the soul to dwell
To the beholder
the Creator breathes in
life's spirit
in that likeness

From the likeness comes
the voice of the Creator
beckoning me near,
but alas!
as nature decrees
I hear close to my ear
an opposing voice,
an adversary,
also hearkening me near

Woe is fate!
between two voices
one must I choose,
but that of
the adversary mocks,
like that of the serpent
who deceives

I stop to ponder . . .
reasoning, I find,
fails to provide me
with more than an "ought"
on which to act

But comes the time
when my highest desire
passes me by
and whets my lips,
I am then obliged
to act on hope

However, what desire
never tarnishes?
So I quicken my search
for another and another,
until I am at wit's end,
without success,
but would I then,
as Abraham,
give hope up entirely—
that is never again
to follow its sweetest
desire—
I might as he, find a
stronger one
With knife in hand,
Abraham raised his arm
and slashed down at his
son
who was bound to an altar,
and in that awesome
moment
there was for him no
turning back, he had
beyond
any doubt given up his
most precious hope, for

ever,
yet paradoxically, he found
it again, for when
it was all over,
Isaac looked up and
smiled

As Abraham sacrificed
Isaac, he simultaneously
sacrificed himself:
he wagered his destiny
on a hope that the act
he was about to carry out
was a command
coming from
an authority higher than
his own

So it was,
by acting without
sufficient reason
one hope's inner authority
Abraham had won
for himself
a greater hope

Abraham achieved
his inner conviction
in 'heroic' dialogue,
however today,
the same conviction
comes through
'living' dialogue:
between oneself
and a fellow being

In 'living' dialogue
I sympathetically feel
the emotions of my fellow
and I build
in my imagination on

them
an experience of my own;
in this way I come to
an 'organic'
understanding
of my reality

Out of understanding
a whole vision comes to
me
and now I am able to
look back and give
relative meaning,
as in a patchwork,
to the "parts"
belonging to the whole
of my reality

By giving meaning
of my own making
to reality,
I empower myself
with a personal belief

By acting on
my own belief
I earn hope enough
to crack the shell
of fear encapsulating me

Now as my final days
draw near,
I stand alone
in front of my own
tribunal in fear
and remorse

However with hope
at hand to subdue
the "Doppleganger"
of fear crouching
at my doorstep,

I am able to face
the ultimate challenge
of living: dying

—Hayim Sholem

After Hayim's death several people wrote to us and shared how peaceful his last days had been. Friends had kept vigil over him and he had not died alone. He was accorded a Jewish burial, and his friends had gathered to pray for him and to say "Shalom."

Hayim knew that there were many aspects of his earlier life that he could not go back and rectify. One cannot make up for what was not given at an earlier time. He did, however, manage to create an authentic existence in his second life and this was quite a feat. Most of us change but seldom do we turn in such a way as to create a wholeness that unites every aspect of our being. Hayim (Life) Sholem (Peace) lived up to his name and left behind hope.

When I was a child, like many children, I loved to throw pebbles into quiet pools of water. The pebble would strike the water and create ripples that far outdistanced the pebble's original entry point. The staff that ministered to Hayim could not have envisioned the effects of their healing care. Hayim never spoke of the technology that helped to keep him alive. He talked about the staff that had helped him to live a life of hope.

Bernard Siegel is a physician who works in partnership with his patients. He is an established, conventionally trained physician who has overcome the limitations of his training while retaining the medically sound principles of his profession. He is not afraid to offer hope to his patients and to bring them into the decision-making process.

Medicine needs to stop trying to fight death, and instead teach people how to live. I think that is really what medicine was founded on . . . Then it isn't so important if you change someone's life or not—that could be up to patients. They could say, "I haven't learned how to live yet. I need two more years to learn about love

and life and sharing, talking to my kids. Please, may I have that."
But patients also have the right to say, "Thank you, no."[3]

Julia was a patient who said "no" to a second round of surgery for cancer and was told by her irate surgeon that she could go home and die then. Initially, a routine physical examination had revealed the possibility of cancer. Diagnostic tests were ordered and the results confirmed that she did have cancer. Surgery was scheduled as soon as possible.

I saw Julia several times before her surgery. We worked on breathing and other calming exercises, as well as an image of healing. She was responsive and very much aware of what was good for her. She was in a private room that accommodated her frequent family visits and had a second bed for the two aunts who alternated staying with her each night. Julia had a loving family and she felt that they were her best medicine.

I went to see Julia a few days after her surgery. She was sitting up in bed and her aunt was lovingly brushing and arranging her hair. She was doing well, but the prognosis was not good. A few days later, I entered her room and she was crying. She said that her surgeon had stated that she must have a second surgery and he wanted the surgery to be performed immediately. She started to sob, but she was able to go on.

> I told him that I need to go home first. I want to walk on the beach and relax for awhile. I want to feel the warmth of the sun and to allow some time to heal from the first surgery. He was very angry when he left my room.

She told me later that his last words to her had been: "Then go home and die."

Julia did go home, but she did not die. She took her beach walks, took some time for relaxation, utilized her tapes, and spent time with her family and friends. Several months later she went through a series of diagnostic tests and there were no signs of her cancer. Two years later she was still doing well. I remember her voice as she described what she needed. She was, I feel, healed by the warmth of the sun, the ocean walks, her loving family, and that which is not so easily explained.

Patients do have a right to make choices, and sometimes they choose possible death over treatment. In Julia's case, she did not rule out the treatment, but she did make a decision to play an active role in the treatment protocol. She trusted her own instincts and she was at peace with her choice. This too enhanced her healing.

It is not easy for patients to make choices because they then have to assume some of the responsibility for the outcome. It is also difficult for some physicians to give up the vertical position of power. Siegel continues:

> Physicians don't want to take no for an answer. Some physicians have literally shouted obscenities when patients have asked about choices . . . I have learned to accept my patients and offer them choices. I find this also makes it easier for them to accept me. We become a healing team.[4]

The majority of patients who seek medical services are not suffering from a discernible organic disorder. They are suffering from disorders that arise from within but most often have to do with their life as a whole. Many of my patients feel out of control, but they do not realize that they, themselves, have the resources to gain a better sense of balance. The first step in healing is to help calm the patient.

> Physicians have to realize that it is treatment to calm somebody, to give hope. It is not unscientific to make somebody feel better.[5]

Siegel's words present a challenge to the healing arts to recognize the power of the human factor in the healing process. When technology and treatment are administered without regard for this factor, the potential for healing is diminished. It is also important to respect those who incorporate this factor into their treatment process. Too often the healing that has gone on between nurses and their patients, social workers and their clients, therapists and their patients, and all others who minister to other people is discounted and/or devalued.

I once sat in on a pain treatment staff meeting, with a hierarchy of one psychiatrist, two clinical psychologists, and three pain therapists. One pain therapist provided a case report and several members of the staff responded. She was an excellent therapist and worked well with her patients. After she had concluded her report, one of the psychologists noted that it was obvious that she spent time talking and listening to her patients. He then stated, "I guess that you provide some of the type of therapy that people traditionally received in barber shops and beauty shops." He liked the therapeutic results, but he did not fully respect the person or the process. What happened during that meeting is what sometimes happens between patients and therapists. The three group members who represented the highest positions in this hierarchy practiced a vertical relationship with their patients and their subordinates. They were addressed by title while patients and subordinates were called by their first names. The psychiatrist spent the least time with the patients, and he mainly addressed their pharmaceutical needs. The psychologists saw most pain patients at least once and sometimes on an irregular basis over a period of time. The pain therapists generally saw most patients at least once a week over an extended period of time. In this particular case, the hierarchy was also both gender- and income-related.

This scenario does not provide maximum benefit for either the patients or the therapists. I believe that the writings of Bernie Siegel as well as numerous other therapists offer an alternative approach that is more conducive to healing.

> The most difficult threat a doctor has to face is that of not being in the protected position of "doctor." I chose to be Bernie Siegel in the hospital—I chose to display the fact that I am a human being. It's much easier to be Dr. Siegel. You have to respect Dr. Siegel, you don't have to respect Bernie. Whatever your profession, it's easier to present yourself in that role than as a human being. To a certain

extent technology has brought this about, and that is why it is a mixed blessing for medicine. It has led doctors away from saying to people, "What happened in your life? . . . I would say 90% of illness—some disease is congenital—but 90% of illness is probably related to something happening in the patient's life.[6]

Siegel makes it clear that he is not saying that the only etiologic factor in illness is the state of one's life, but he does emphasize the relationship between illness and one's past life. He also makes it clear that it is not a matter of blaming the patient, but rather of saying that the patient has participated in the illness. "The healing process demands that patients know who they were so they know who to become."

It is important for therapists to acknowledge their own pain. This does not mean that we turn to the patient for healing, but rather that we meet that patient and acknowledge their pain. D. Jesse Peters states:

> If we have faced our own pain, if we are not afraid to feel it, we will be able to face the patient in all of his or her pain. And through this act, a connection is made which has the power to transcend any disease. We acknowledge a primary reality which we both share and over which we have limited control. We give legitimacy to the struggle, and thereby give hope that recovery is possible.[7]

One of my patients called me an appropriate guide. I felt that this was a great compliment. She had often come into my office expressing feelings of despair. She felt psychologically and physically wounded and had daily headaches that were often severe enough to completely restrict her daily activities. She lived a fragile existence that seemed forever in danger of collapsing. There were times when I was amazed that she had kept her appointment. In time, however, I could sense moments of strength. She was beginning to set some limits and to express her own needs. Her headaches diminished, and there were longer periods of being able to accomplish minimum daily tasks. Sometimes, she would express her anger and I could see a toughness that had been a big part of her earlier years. It was this toughness that had been used to hide her vulnerabilities. She had kept her emotions and her pain well hidden for many years. When, however, she sustained a shoulder/neck injury that led to the loss of her job, her whole life was suddenly thrown into chaos. She lost her financial independence; she had to give up her apartment and move into a room; and she felt rejected by her former co-workers. She was newly injured, but many of her old wounds that had never fully healed were now a renewed source of pain.

The first time we met for pain therapy I had called her by her given name of Barbara. She had not corrected me, but several sessions later she told me that she liked to be called Bobbie. I felt that we had moved beyond the initial stage of protected formality. During our pain therapy sessions we worked on calming exercises, self-regulation skills, pain management, autogenics, and guided imagery. She began to tell me what was working and what was not working for her. She was beginning to share in the responsibility for her treatment program, but there was no demand to do so. We discussed her symptoms, her family, her former workplace, and her needs. We explored past resources and looked for new ones. We worked in partnership and tried to avoid the dependence that sometimes develops over time. Her strength would come from recreating a future, and she needed both support and a sense of freedom to accomplish this goal. She was entering new territory and it was an honor to be her guide. Now and then, she expressed hope in the future and I shared with her this sense of hope. Howard Stein states:

> The subject of medicine is life, not disease . . . What life is about: the struggle to balance often irreconcilable conflicts; the experience of love, suffering, joy, loss, hope, despair, anxiety. Often we give prescriptions, or urge them on our patients, when what both we and they need is something much more slowly acquired, insight into life . . . We need to conduct our therapeutic communication and intervention strategies with our ear attuned to the developmental process underlying sickness and health that is "speaking" to us through the pathology—if we have only the courage to listen . . . To say "Thou" to a patient, and mean it, one must be able

to utter "I" to oneself. One can then stand with his patient, because he can stand alone with himself. This is the essence of medicine, of therapeutic communication, of life.[8]

Notes

1. Norman Cousins, "State of mind does affect state of health," *Los Angeles Times* (July 10, 1985), sec. II, p. 5.
2. Hayim Sholem, *Hope: My Response to Dying* (Jerusalem, Israel, 1987).
3. Bernard Siegel, "The health of the healing professions: An interview with Bernard Siegel," *Revision*, Vol. 7, No. 1 (Spring, 1984), p. 87.
4. Ibid., p. 88.
5. Ibid., p. 89.
6. Ibid., p. 92.
7. Dr. Jesse Peters, Editorial: "Acknowledging Pain," *Stanford Medical School Student Journal*, 1990.
8. Howard Stein, "Toward a life of dialogue: Therapeutic communication and the meaning of medicine," *Continuing Education for the Family Physician* (April 1982), pp. 29–30, 32, 37, 44–45.

CHAPTER 13

Maintaining an Image of Well Being

Maintaining an image of well being is not easy when one has to contend with daily pain, but Margo makes this effort every day of her life. I mentioned Margo in the first chapter of this book, and I am pleased to reintroduce her in this chapter. After the completion of her pain therapy program, we had discussed having lunch in one year. She was in the process of moving to Southern California, and I was living abroad for the year. I gave her my home telephone number and looked forward to hearing from her. Two years passed before I once again heard from Margo, and it was a welcome call. I learned that she had misplaced my telephone number and had been unable to obtain the number from my former workplace. She had, however, come across it while she was unpacking some books and papers. We made our luncheon appointment. Now that it was over two years since I had seen her I hoped, as one does when there is a lapse of time, that I would easily recognize her among the many people at the restaurant. I did recognize her, standing there with her excellent posture and looking lovely and well groomed. It did not take long to close the gap of time, and we found that we needed more time in which to talk than one lunch would afford. We did not discuss Margo's pain, but I was aware that her image of well being was very much a personal effort. During this first meeting, I asked Margo if she would be willing to add her voice to this book. She agreed to do so, and I thank her for sharing her courage and her efforts to establish and maintain a sense of well being.

Margo

Before I was referred for biofeedback/pain therapy I had tried everything imaginable. I had traveled to a medical clinic in the Northeast and to one in the Southeast. I had completed a pain program for my back discomfort and one for the rehabilitation of my neck muscles. I had sought psychological help, and I had also tried to find a support group. I even tried to form my own support group, and we met for a brief time in my home. The only support groups in my community were ones for drug addiction and alcoholism. There was nothing for chronic pain, and I did not know where to turn.

I decided to go to a clinic located in Southern California. My husband and I had been thinking of moving to this area, and we decided to combine my treatment with some house hunting. I was currently suffering from daily neck, shoulder, and back pain, but my primary complaint, at this time, was the itching, burning, and acute sensitivity of my upper legs and the postsurgical pelvic pain.

During my first week at the clinic I was seen by one doctor after another and then I was referred to the pain treatment center. I was given a psychological test, met with a psychologist, and was then referred for biofeedback/pain therapy. The psychologist seemed to feel that the biofeedback would help me, but what really helped me was the pain therapist. She not only helped my physically, but she also helped me mentally. She gave me the rapport that I needed, and she also gave me warmth and caring. She listened, and I felt that I was making progress. Because of her I wanted to return for additional sessions, but first I had to go home and take care of some personal business.

While I was gone my husband rented a home in a retirement community. We decided to "test the waters" before making our final decision about moving, and I would complete my treatment program during this time. In due course, these treatments and my husband's care and support helped me, more than any of the medications helped me, so that today I find that I am living a more useful life.

When I was told to start biofeedback, I felt very resistant to it mentally. However, since nothing else had helped me, I felt I might as well give this a try as well. I had nothing more to lose and maybe something to gain. The biofeedback treatment helped me to learn how to relax, and in learning how to relax it helped me to cope with things in a much easier way. But the main thing that I got out of the entire treatment was my therapist. She's the one that really helped me understand that it isn't always the mechanisms and medication that is given to you that helps. It's the understanding and the empathy that you feel towards someone. That helped me more than anything, so much so that I looked forward to each session instead of dreading it. The biofeedback and the help that I got from my therapist helped me see things more clearly. When you begin to see things more clearly, it's as if a weight is lifted, and when the pain starts to minimize, it's as if a whole new world begins to open up for you. You see everything so differently, and you can cope with things and you can weigh them and look at them objectively, whereas before everything was focused on me, myself, and I.

While I was preparing for the first trip to the Southern California clinic, I did not know what awaited me, and I couldn't pack. I had clothes hanging up, but I could not make a decision about anything. My hands were shaking. I couldn't eat. I couldn't even decide what to eat for dinner or lunch. Decisions were passé; I just could not make them. I just couldn't think beyond my pain. Before the treatment I was totally dependent on my husband. In retrospect, I think that a lesser man might have left me. Sometimes I would just lie in bed. Sometimes I couldn't even select a television station. I think I was either on the verge of a nervous breakdown or in the midst of a nervous breakdown. I will never really know, and how I made it out to California I will never know. It was so terrible that if we went anywhere, and I had to meet someone, I would have to take a change of clothes in the car. I would wear casual comfortable clothes so that I could lie down in the back seat of the car and rest. When we neared our destination we would find a place for me to change my clothes, so that I would be more appropriately dressed. There were many times when I promised to do something, and then backed out at the last moment. My whole life was ruled by my pain.

Shortly before leaving for California I saw a prominent endocrinologist. He told me that I had hyperparathyroidism, and that this condition accounted for most of my pain and some of my other symptoms. He wanted to operate immediately, but when I told him that I was scheduled to go to a clinic in California, he suggested a second opinion at that institution. I felt, at that time, that I finally knew the source of my illness, but the next specialist told me that while I did have the condition, he preferred to treat it with medication and to check me from time to time. I am still on the medication, and there are no plans for a surgery.

My real problems began, I think, I know they began in 1976. I was helping my husband in his business, and I was running my own business. I was under a great deal of stress, and one night, as I was driving home from work, a fast-moving car hit my car. It was a terrible accident, and I was severely injured. I had to have head and neck surgery, but as soon as I could, I went back to work. I continued to work until my back went out in 1982. At that point I began my search for some help. I had acupuncture, nerve blocks, physical therapy, heat and cold packs, medications, and many medical consultations. Finally, in 1983, I had a laminectomy. I had a microlaminectomy, which I was told later had not been done correctly. I was, however, coping fairly well until I had two successive falls. My first fall came at a time when I was preparing for a family trip. I was hurrying down our porch stairs and fell and broke my ankle. My foot and lower leg were in a cast for ten weeks, and during that time I fell again and fractured several ribs. This was a low point in my life, and I even had thoughts of suicide. My injuries and walking with a cast on my foot and leg caused additional strain on my back. I felt helpless and hopeless, but somehow I was able to pull out of it. My husband was supportive, as always, and he helped care for me during this difficult time. To this day I suffer from all of these previous injuries. All of my later symptoms, and especially the pelvic discomfort, just added more pain to my previous chronic-pain state.

I was asked how I happened to make some major changes in my life, and how I mustered the courage to confront so many aspects of my life at a time when I had a great deal of pain to deal with. I don't really know, except I knew that if I did not change my life, at this point, I would become stagnant, and I would keep going downhill. We had rented at a place in a retirement community, and I realized that here was a way of life that would give me comfort. If anything were to happen to my husband, I would have enough to keep me busy, enough to confront me, enough to go on with my life, and a chance for happiness. I also had family members in the area and the beginnings of some new friendships. My new physical therapist had changed my outlook on life, and I trusted my current physicians. Most of all I was relating to a life outside of my own problems and my pain, but still I was very torn by this decision. It was difficult to think of leaving my elderly mother alone in another state, but she was not willing or well enough to leave at this time. I knew that she would never forgive me for leaving, and she never did. My husband was also ill, and I was afraid that this might be our last chance to create a new life together. I felt that if I stayed where I was, I would become a vegetable.

I was in a great deal of pain, which I am every single day, but somehow knowing that my life would be changed gave me a new perspective, and I could deal with the pain better than I had at any other time. I went back home, and I alone started getting the ball rolling for the move. My husband stayed behind and readied the new home that we had purchased. How I did it, I don't ever know, but somehow you're given added strength when the mind wants to do something so badly that it even overcomes the pain. My mother became very ill after I returned home and was not expected to live. I thought maybe the decision to leave would be made easier. My mother lived, however, and my husband stayed out in California for several months getting things lined up in our new house. I sat for almost two months in a hospital with my mother, thinking she wouldn't come home. But after Christmas she did come home, and I had to get her an around-the-clock nurse. Because I was trying to do so much, and because this conflict was so difficult for me, naturally the pain increased, but I was determined not to let it get the better of me. I coped as best I could, but I did look for another biofeedback/pain therapist. I could not find one that could help me as my former therapist had, so I finally ended up relying on what I had already learned.

Margo had made life-affirming choices that necessitated facing her own needs. She had spent a lifetime trying to please others, especially her mother. She had routinely silenced her own voice, and now she knew that she was in danger of spending the rest of her life much as she had spent most of her adult years. She needed to give herself permission to live her own life, and that was exactly what she did. Her image of well being is based on this courage.

Margo's treatment for chronic pain illustrates how difficult it is to provide effective treatment for chronic-pain patients, and how desperate patients become in their search for relief from their pain. During my training in Integral Medicine, I worked with both the theoretical and clinical aspects of pain treatment and for a short period of time I observed and participated in the UCLA Pain Control Unit. David Bresler was the director. I did not realize, at the time, how unique this pain treatment center was. Richard Trubo, in his introductory remarks to the book that he and David Bresler wrote, states:

> As part of the prestigious UCLA Medical Center, the Pain Control Unit occupies a section of the bottom floor of a large university building. Its operations are far from glamorous—an overworked staff, cramped offices, and aging furniture. But despite such obstacles, its pain alleviation program has been quietly prospering with relatively little public notice . . . I met people, young and old, who had spent months and years hobbling from one doctor to another, frustrated in their search for pain relief. They had tried all the wonder drugs, and miracle surgeries, with little more to show for it than the complications often associated with these chemical and surgical assaults on the body . . . Interestingly, many of these patients were initially as skeptical of the Pain Control Unit's program as I was. They were referred there by personal physicians who were often convinced they were beyond help. These patients had been told that probably nothing could ever help ease the terrible, chronic pain in their head, neck, arms, or back. So how, they asked, after futilely trying the most sophisticated pain-alleviation techniques that Western medicine can offer, could these new approaches be any help at all?[1]

Trubo interviewed many of the Pain Control Unit patients, and he was surprised to find that the patients did improve. This low-budget, outpatient clinic demonstrated that few chronic-pain patients are beyond help, but as far as I know, the Pain Control Unit never managed to move beyond being an experimental program in a basement location. It no longer exists at UCLA, but the well-known traditional pain treatment center does still exist. Here the emphasis is on pharmacology, surgical intervention, and research. The closure of the UCLA Pain Control Unit was a loss to the community and to all of the patients who might have benefited from this fine program.

In his book *Free Yourself From Pain*, Bresler states:

> The UCLA Pain Control Unit was established on the premise that every pain patient who truly wants to get better can be helped to at least some degree, regardless of the prognosis of conventional medicine. This basic supposition has yet to be refuted. The key to our success lies in the creation of a treatment program individualized to each patient. Such a program may include ancient techniques like acupuncture or yoga, as well as more modern forms of therapy, such as biofeedback and ultrasonic stimulation. Although we prefer to use the most noninvasive and natural approaches whenever possible, we do utilize drugs or nerve blocks when we feel that they are more appropriate. And how do we determine what's most appropriate? By getting to know as much as we can about each patient's unique life situation, and by enlisting the active cooperation of patients in the development of their own therapeutic programs.[2]

Bresler, in the first chapter of his book, summarizes some of his personal conclusions about the nature of chronic pain. He states:

All Pain Is Real

The pain experience involves a complex interaction of physical, mental, and spiritual factors ... Pain is an intense personal experience, and even if a doctor can find no physical reason for your pain, it is still real.

Pain Is a Positive Message

Chronic pain is usually not a disease or mistake; rather it is a symptom generated through the wisdom of the body. In my opinion, symptoms are the way that the body tries to heal itself or prevent further injury. Once their message is heard and appropriate action taken, symptoms will usually disappear, for they are no longer needed.

Effective Therapy Is Most Seriously Blocked by Unrealistic Beliefs and Expectations

If a doctor has ever told you, "I'm sorry, but there's nothing more that can be done for you," you probably found it devastating . . . By declaring your case hopeless, he has given you the negative and unrealistic expectation that you must live with pain for the rest of your life . . . How you see your reality affects how you experience it.

The Mind Is the Safest and Most Powerful Pain Reliever

Anyone who has studied psychology is aware of the untapped potential of the mind . . . biofeedback and guided imagery clearly demonstrate the power of the mind.

Self-Control Is the Key to Achieving Long-Lasting Relief

With diligent practice, you can learn to relax yourself on command, even in the face of overwhelming stress. By eating more nutritious foods, you can provide your body with the essential materials needed to activate its inner pain control system and to maximize its self-healing potential . . . Certain self-control techniques, such as relaxation and guided imagery, may involve the endorphin system or some other physiological mechanisms yet to be discovered. What is important is that you may be able to do more than anyone else to overcome your discomfort.

No Pain Problem Is Hopeless

In talking to thousands of people with pain in recent years, I've concluded that their "hopeless" state of mind has often been aggravated because they've attempted to smother pain's symptoms instead of trying to understand pain's message—from a physical, mental, emotional, and spiritual viewpoint . . . [Only with this understanding] can long-lasting improvement in your condition occur. And it will. Your situation is not hopeless. But I wonder how many lives have been wasted because patients have been convinced that "nothing more can be done."[3]

The UCLA Pain Control Unit provided me with an opportunity to observe and participate in a patient program that united the theory and practice of Integral Medicine. I observed the benefits of a varied, but integrated patient treatment program. I feel privileged that Carol Wilson allowed me to observe her patient education classes, and I also benefited from my participation in other aspects of this very effective outpatient-treatment program. Patients and staff members were treated with respect, and there was ample support for the patients, as they learned to assume some of the responsibility for their own treatment choices.

Many of the patients being treated at the Pain Control Unit had been considered poor candidates for improvement, and most were very disabled by their chronic-pain symptoms. Like Margo, most had also been through multiple pain programs and had obtained only limited results. The patients in the Pain Control Unit did improve, and what, you might ask, made the difference? There were, of course, many factors, but I believe that the patient needs to feel involved in what I call a reasonable partnership. He/she needs to have the opportunity to make choices and to be held accountable for a reasonable level of participation. The inclusion of alternative treatment modalities presents a wider range of treatment choices. Many traditional pain treatment programs have fixed programs that are limited in scope. Acupuncture, acupressure, massage, dance therapy, yoga, and certain other "hands-on techniques" greatly enhance the treatment program.

A major topic in this book is the healing partnership, and this is possibly the most important factor in an effective treatment program. Too often mutual respect is lacking, and patients and therapists become adversaries. Each one views the other with mistrust, and both parties are set up for failure.

In the healing partnership the therapist acknowledges and nurtures the patient's own resources while giving the patient credit for his or her coping skills. The patient's image of well being may develop within the meeting between the therapist and the patient, but it is important for the patient to strengthen this image from within his or her own community. When a therapist encourages dependency, the patient's image of wellness is a fragile one.

The patient and the therapist are, in the best sense, teachers to each other. I learned from Margo that maintaining an image of well being is a lifelong task that cannot be taken for granted but must be forged out of the everyday. What first struck me about Margo was her sense of humor and the fact that despite her pain, her inner child was alive and well. She has passion, and she applies herself to the present. Margo needs to guard against her tendency to be a perfectionist, and she strives to set limits on her expectations of herself and others. She is not perfect, and she has learned to forgive her imperfections. She is honest, and she shares her humanity. She presents a beautiful image, and she is that image.

There are some people, like Cindy, who do not have the resources to maintain an image of well being. I see her on an irregular basis, but when she makes an appointment she keeps it. She is presently living on welfare, and she trades housework for a place to live. For a short time she lived in her car, and she has not had a stable home for two years. There was a time when she had a well-paying job, custody of her two children, and her own home. Her children now live with their father, and she feels sad when she sees them. They are understanding, but it does not relieve her pain. She has daily pain from a back injury, but she is more emotionally injured than physically disabled.

Cindy comes to me to talk and to spend some quiet time listening to a meditative tape. She is very verbal about what type of tapes are most helpful, and she utilizes the practice tapes that I have given her. She does not want sympathy; she wants to be heard, and she needs to keep her sense of dignity intact. Cindy is a survivor, and while I do make professional suggestions I know that meeting her daily survival needs must be her main priority.

Cindy's image of well being was shattered over a period of time, but there is also a life history that has served to limit her resources. When I see Cindy we discuss ways to decrease her pain, but it is the daily assaults upon her dignity that currently undermine her ability to reestablish an image of well being. She does, however, have courage, and she is attempting to rebuild her world. The last time I saw her I shared this Hasidic Tale.

True Sorrow and True Joy

When he was asked which was the right way, that of sorrow or that of joy, the rabbi of Berditchev said, "There are two kinds of sorrow and two kinds of joy. When a man broods over the misfortunes that have come upon him, when he cowers in a corner and despairs of help—that is a bad kind of sorrow, concerning which it is said: 'The Divine Presence does not dwell in a place of dejection.' The other kind is the honest grief of a man who knows what he lacks. The same is true of joy. He who is devoid of inner substance, and, in the midst of his empty pleasures, does not feel it, nor tries to fill his lack, is a fool. But he who is truly joyful is like a man whose house has burned down, who feels his need deep in his soul and begins to build anew. Over every stone that is laid, his heart rejoices."[4]

Notes

1. David Bresler, *Free Yourself from Pain* (New York: Simon and Schuster, 1979), pp. 13–14.
2. Ibid., pp. 24–25.
3. Ibid., pp. 25–30.
4. Martin Buber, *Tales of the Hasidim: The Early Masters* (New York: Shocken Books, 1946), p. 226.

CHAPTER 14

The Patient as VIP

My mother's youngest sister, 14-year-old Ruthie Hulpher, suffered from chronic stomach aches. In 1933, her symptoms worsened and reached an acute stage of discomfort. She was rushed to the nearest medical facility but they refused to treat her. Her family was referred to a county facility that was 50 miles away. This facility, which still exists today, was one of the few hospitals that provided emergency care for the poor. By the time Ruthie's condition was accurately diagnosed and treated she was beyond medical help. Her chronic appendicitis had been ignored for years, and now the accumulation of toxic materials had spilled over and contaminated her whole body. The family kept a vigil during the five days that preceded her death, and each mourned for many years the void that her death created. Poverty and ignorance were vectors that contributed to her death. Ruthie's mother cared about her eight children, but she was a widow, and she barely earned enough to provide shelter and food for her children. Obtaining medical care for a child with chronic "stomach aches" was looked upon as a luxury that she could not afford.

In 1964, my 4-year-old son, Ken, sustained an eye injury while on a Sunday outing in a country recreational area. I rushed him to the closest emergency facility, and he was given treatment as soon as possible. The waiting room was filled with crying babies, restless children, and ill and injured people of all ages. During our hourlong wait for service, ambulances arrived and delivered still more patients to this overburdened emergency facility.

The attending physician examined my son's injured eye and recommended that I take him home and call his pediatrician in the morning. I was not comfortable with this prescription so I called his pediatrician from the emergency room. He made arrangements for my son to see an eye specialist that very evening. I drove the 50 miles into the city, met with the eye specialist, and soon my son, who was now in a state of shock, was hospitalized and being treated for his eye injury. The next day the physician stated that a delay in his treatment would have caused permanent blindness in the injured eye.

I was fortunate because I had health insurance that made it possible for me to demand better-quality medical treatment for my son. I also recognized the seriousness of his injury, even when the attending physician had failed to do so. I have often wondered how many of the people that I sat with in that crowded waiting room were simply sent home to nurse themselves or to nurse as best they could their injured or ill children.

Emergency treatment for the severely injured or those who are gravely ill has improved over the years, but there are ever-increasing numbers of people who have only limited access to a health system that provides basic health care. Without cash or medical insurance, many treatable maladies go untreated. Even when medical insurance is available, there are often clauses that exclude the treatment of pre-existing conditions or severely limit the treatment protocol.

Having medical insurance enhances the possibilities of obtaining adequate medical care, but excellent health care individualizes the treatment program and focuses on both the patient's current health needs and preventive medicine. This type of medical treatment is too often limited to the designated VIPs (very important patients).

I once worked at a medical clinic that designated wealthy donors or potential donors as VIPs. I did give these patients excellent care, but when asked if I had done so, I replied that, as far as I am concerned, all of my patients were VIPs. Of course, I did know the difference. VIPs knew that they deserved excellent health and they had the means to demand the best. Everyone deserves excellent health care, but many people have been deprived of even the most basic health care. When this occurs, there is an ever-increasing number of people who are likely to develop chronic disorders.

Walt was a designated VIP. He was a contributor to the institution, and he had an economic base that might well provide additional contributions in the future. Once a year, he participated in a comprehensive executive health program, and at age 65 Walt's health was excellent. There had, however, been a recent increase in his blood-pressure levels and a course in biofeedback therapy was recommended.

From the first moment that I met Walt, it was apparent that he liked to be in control. He had a no-nonsense approach laced with a spirit of enthusiasm. It was also apparent that he was accustomed to success, and he was confident that he could manage his elevated blood-pressure levels as well as he managed the rest of his life. During our initial sessions together I covered basic stress-management techniques, and utilized a constant-cuff, blood-pressure, biofeedback device to demonstrate how the blood-pressure readings decreased during times of quiet meditation and relaxed breathing. During our third session Walt stated that he wanted to tell me about the best physician that he had ever encountered.

Mike was my physician, and a social friend, for some years. About five years ago he noticed that my blood-pressure levels were elevated, and he suggested that I pick one of the two treatment programs that he had to offer. I could either take medications or I could join his exercise program. If I joined his program, I would have to make a commitment to walk two times per week, for one hour, at an appointed time. Other issues were also addressed, but this was the heart of the program. If I decided to take the medications, I would be charged for all office calls, and my blood pressure would be monitored on a weekly basis. If I joined the exercise group, I would have to put up $5000 and stay in the program for six months. If, at the end of the six-month period, my blood-pressure levels were back to normal, I would be able to designate what charitable organization to which I wanted my money to be donated. If I dropped out of the program or failed to decrease my blood-pressure levels, the money would go to Mike. For six months I took my twice-weekly morning walks, and Mike set a brisk pace. We were a group of four, and at the end of each week we had a short discussion about other aspects of our treatment program. I had my blood pressure monitored on a weekly basis. By the end of the fourth month my blood-pressure levels were consistently within a normal range. By the end of the program I was feeling great, and so was one of my favorite charities.

For the next three years I walked on a regular basis. What really helped me was seeing Mike at our various social gatherings. Seeing him kept me on track, but then he retired and moved to another area. During the last year and a half I have slipped, but now I am ready to get back on track.

During our time together Walt had mentioned increased concerns about his wife's health and other stressors in his life, but he was uncomfortable when the conversation turned to personal issues. I did not push him, but I did reinforce his basic capacity to evaluate a problem and do something about it.

Walt completed two more treatment sessions. In one sense he had rediscovered what he already knew, but he had also developed additional resources. Walt stated: "I'm living proof that you *can* teach an old dog some new tricks. I've benefited from this program. I've had some good teachers along the way and I thank you for being one of them."

Walt deserved the excellent health care that he had come to expect, but medicine that caters to the affluent does not offer excellent health care. Excellence is not just a matter of advanced technology; it is the treatment of individuals. Impersonal care is demeaning. Excellent health care may go beyond the confines of an office space or a traditional treatment program, but in all cases the patient is viewed as a VIP.

I have been treated by many physicians over the years, but

one stands out. I was not ill when I contacted her office for an appointment. I wanted her input about maintaining my health, and I had some personal health-related questions to discuss. I was given an appointment date, and a packet of materials and questionnaires were sent to my home. I filled out all of the necessary information and mailed it back to the office. On the day of my appointment I arrived at the specified time and was shown a preappointment video. The video was designed for patient education, and I was beginning to wonder when I would finally meet the physician. Shortly after the video had ended I was ushered into her office. It was not exactly an office, but rather a combination office/workspace that was comfortable and inviting. She had a family practice and informed me that she now specialized in promoting wellness and not in curing illness. We had a 70-minute conversation and a minimal physical examination. She listened to my questions, and she answered them in a simple, direct manner. I only remember two items. In response to my question about a healthy diet, she suggested eating a variety of foods but especially to select those foods that were in season. Toward the end of our conversation she noted that much of my life had been spent nurturing others and that I should consider writing or some other avenues to develop my own creativity. Here was a physician who was addressing me in a way that no other physician ever had. Immediately, she had seemed to sense my needs. Her words did not have an immediate impact on my life, but what had transpired during our meeting did have an increased meaning over time. To be addressed personally is, in itself, very meaningful.

I am fond of a quote which I first came across in the writings of David Bresler:

> The ancient Chinese distinguished five levels of physicians. Lowest was the veterinarian or animal doctor. Next came the doctor who used acupuncture, moxibustion, herbs and other procedures for relieving specific complaints. Third was the surgeon, who treated more serious problems. Second highest was the nutritionist, who practiced the "medicine of longevity" by teaching what to eat. Highest of all was the philosopher–doctor, or Sage, who taught

people the order of the universe. The Sage is the only doctor who can effect a genuine cure, for he treats directly by going right to the cause of the illness: the patient's ignorance of how to live harmoniously with nature.

Excellent health care also serves to educate the patient. Ignorance can be cured. Most of the chronic-pain patients whom I see have very little understanding of what may be serving to exacerbate their symptoms. When they gain basic understanding regarding their condition, they begin to see that they share in the responsibility for improving and/or maintaining their health. Technology provides valuable information, but education is best served when one human being reaches out to another and addresses his or her needs.

Marian

Marian had managed her chronic back pain for several years, but when the symptoms began to worsen she consulted her personal physician. The physician examined her and referred her to an orthopedic surgeon. Marian completed a series of diagnostic tests, and the results of this testing showed spinal abnormalities that were related to osteoporosis. The orthopedic surgeon ordered a series of spinal injections that were aimed at decreasing the level of pain. The results of these injections were minimal, and a consultation meeting was scheduled.

The orthopedic surgeon presented Marian with two alternatives. She was advised that she could learn to live with the pain or she could elect to have surgical intervention. He could not guarantee that the surgery would alleviate her pain, but he emphasized that without surgery she might be in a wheelchair within one year. The image of herself in a wheelchair was frightening, and Marian chose to have the surgery.

According to a recent edition of *Vital Times*, a hospital health-care bulletin, "back pain is second only to the common cold as a reason for people seeing their doctors." The article goes on to say that

> Surgical correction is rarely the solution for most back pain suf-
> ferers. In fact, before surgery will be even considered an option, all
> other conservative approaches must have failed to bring relief . . .
> Sometimes surgery eliminates or reduces pain, sometimes it
> doesn't. That is why it is explored only after all other less drastic
> options have been explored.[1]

Marian had been offered only minimal treatment options, and
surgery was presented as the surgeon's treatment of choice. Marian had, during her lifetime, relied on traditional medical treatment, and she trusted the advice of her orthopedic surgeon. In one
sense, she was being treated as a VIP. She had excellent health
coverage, and she was being offered an operation that few people
suffering from chronic back pain could afford. She had never
thought to question the advice of her surgeon, and she had never
explored alternative treatment programs. Marian's back surgery
and posttreatment program cost in excess of $32,000. Her lower
back was fused together, and stabilizing rods were inserted to
brace the spine.

Marian was a compliant patient, and she carefully followed
her physician's postsurgical treatment instructions. She had several adverse reactions to the medications that were initially prescribed for her, but the doses were adjusted, and she did well. One
year after her back surgery Marian was released by her orthopedic
surgeon. He told her that the surgery had been successful. She
reminded him that without medication she had daily lower-back
pain. He stated that she would need to learn to manage her pain
without medication. He had, in his words, done all that he could
do for her, and he wished her well.

For the first time in her life Marian began to explore the
possibility of a nontraditional treatment program. She had decided that she needed a supportive program that would address
her chronic body stiffness, upper-back soreness, and her daily
lower-back pain. With the help of her husband, she found a program that would accept her insurance and offered a personalized
treatment program. She made an appointment at a Center of Natural Medicine. She was soon introduced to acupuncture, acupressure, medical massage, herbs, nutrition, physical exercise, and

a computer diagnosis. She was, in the fullest sense, treated as a VIP. The element of personal uniqueness was fully addressed, and Marian's treatment program was designed to meet her needs. She is currently involved in a comprehensive treatment program, but at all times her own input is valued and respected. As usual, Marian is a compliant patient, and she is beginning to experience the benefits of her treatment program. Soon she will be tapering off the frequency of her treatment sessions, but she realizes that she may benefit from an ongoing maintenance program.

Medicine is more than what you do to a person. It also involves the interaction between the patient and the therapist. When Marian arrives for her current treatments, she is warmly greeted by the office staff. For the first time in her life she is on a first-name basis with her medical therapist, and she enjoys their exchanges during her 90-minute meeting times. The therapist is an important part of the program, but Marian is also receiving a self-help educational program that will help to sustain her when she is seen on a less frequent basis.

Marian states that she has improved since starting her natural-program. "I no longer have upper-back soreness, and I have much less lower-back pain. I do feel stiff in the morning, but my daily walks help to decrease the stiffness." She does not complain about not having a significant improvement after her back surgery.

> Before my surgery I had neck pain and that was completely gone after the surgery. I would recommend that one be sure that back surgery is really necessary, and I would never want to have another back surgery before trying alternative treatments. What is strange about the results of the back surgery is that I had lower-back surgery and my neck pain was cured, but not my lower-back pain.
>
> I'm not sure that I like having the rods in my back, and I still wonder if I really needed them. Basically, I don't dwell on the surgery, but I am thankful that I have both traditional and nontraditional methods to turn to. Right now the nontraditional methods seem to be best for me, but each problem has to be evaluated individually.

When I asked Marian what had helped her to endure her pain, she stated that her daily meditative prayers calmed her fears and provided solace. Her spirituality continues to be a very meaningful part of her life stance.

I once suggested biofeedback-assisted pain therapy to Marian, but after a brief discussion she decided that it was not what she wanted. She was not rejecting help; she simply felt that this was not the help that she needed. The therapist may believe that he or she can help the patient, but this cannot be accomplished without the support and belief of the patient. It is not healthy to deny one's own symptoms, but it is healthy to question which type of treatment is best suited to one's particular health needs.

When the patient is treated as a VIP, he or she is given the opportunity to make decisions. Excellent medical treatment acknowledges the uniqueness of the person being treated and addresses his or her needs. Every patient deserves VIP treatment, but many are not so fortunate as Marian. It is easy to blame patients for their own lack of adequate treatment, but, for many people, the cost of health insurance is simply beyond their means. (I, as well as other health professionals, seldom see people who do not have personal health insurance or who are not being covered under worker's compensation insurance.) This means that many children are denied adequate medical treatment. There is also a fear factor that often goes unaddressed. People from other cultures or those who have been generally kept out of the medical system may fear traditional medical practices. Education and preventive medicine help to prevent the spread of chronic disorders. When one has little choice but to suffer, one's pain may become the only way to express one's chronic suffering.

Notes

1. "Backache and what to do about it," _Vital Times_ (La Jolla: Scripps Memorial Hospitals), p. 4.

CHAPTER 15

Pain Management

Bill Wilson, a former pain-therapy patient, recently stated that he doubts that most people who write about pain management are themselves suffering from chronic pain. I think that he is probably right, and for that reason I have asked Bill and two other patients to share with us their own stories and how they have learned to manage their pain.

Bill is a man who might have stepped out of the Larry McMurtry novel *Lonesome Dove*. He has a quiet strength that does not fully disguise an undercurrent of rage and frustration that may have been fed by any number of past insults and various tributaries of pain that have flown into the present. Bill seems to be a man who had to earn his manhood through rites of passage that continually challenged his survival skills. These survival skills sustained his position among men, but they did not help him to cope with his daily chronic pain.

Bill mentions below that he is not highly educated, but his intelligence and sensitivity cut through to the very essence of pain management. Pain management is an individual journey that can be shared, but it demands a personal response from each chronic-pain sufferer. He also mentions that most of the books that he has read imply that self-help cures are not miracles. I think, however, that people like Bill redefine the word miracle. They are open to the possibility of another reality, and they help to create this reality. Small children take very little for granted. They see miracles in the everyday, and it is the adult world that eventually dims their view. Bill is not better because of a miracle. He is part of the miracle that allows us to repair, to change, and to make choices that affirm life.

Bill

My name is William B. Wilson. I'm a 51-year-old male Caucasian, insulin-dependent diabetic. In July of 1988 I slipped and fell, injuring my lower back. This is a brief explanation of my experience with biofeedback-assisted pain therapy.

After completing a series of medical and psychiatric examinations, I was given a referral for biofeedback-therapy. In the beginning, I did not really have much hope that this was a workable thing for me because I had never experienced it and had no knowledge at all of what was trying to be accomplished. But, with the expert guidance of the pain therapist, I began to understand that if I could accomplish what was being asked of me, there was a possibility that I would be able to control my pain and a lot of my emotional problems. I had a total of 33 sessions of pain therapy. The last twenty or so were with Aleene, which were, I believe, the most beneficial of all because she is a lady of my generation and seems to understand the life experiences and problems that we have when we get into middle age. The system seems to work better when you are working with someone of your own age, and in my case, of the female gender. Man to man, you seem to have a built-in defense system that's very hard to break down. With Aleene, I felt more relaxed and more able to communicate and to receive and digest the information that she was giving me.

One of the first things I learned to do in my treatment program was to change the temperature in my fingers through concentration. I could start a tingling sensation in my feet and bring that sensation up into my arms and fingers. Then I learned that, to a small degree, I could change my heart rate. It was fascinating that I could do this without any medication or anything, but just strictly by my concentration and my thoughts. So, I began to realize that

this was a very serious and beneficial treatment program. I purchased, and was loaned by doctors and other personnel, books
pertaining to the healing of the mind, concentration, and imagery.
These books were by Dr. Bernie Siegel, Dr. Sobel, Dr. Norman
Cousins of UCLA, and many others who I do not, at this time,
recall. I read a total of 12 or 13 fairly good-sized books pertaining
to this subject. I have also acquired a tape library of approximately
50 biofeedback tapes, many of which are subliminal.

You can help yourself. These tapes are very valuable to your
recovery if you will be open-minded, let your defenses down, and
try to listen, not just hear. It's very important that you want to listen
and that you listen to a tape over and over again, because, in my
opinion, a one-time thing is of no benefit. It takes many, many
times of listening to the same tape and of concentrating on it to
really benefit from the message. Each time you will hear different
messages and different words. You will soon be able to isolate
yourself from your surroundings, and concentrate entirely on the
tape. One important factor is that you must learn to utilize the
outside sounds, such as traffic or telephones ringing, or some other
distractions, to enhance your concentration, not to disturb it. In my
earlier attempts to practice and to concentrate I would become very
irritable and disturbed when the phone would ring or a car horn
would blow. But with the assistance and guidance of Dr. Figueroa
at the clinic, I was able to utilize these sounds to deepen my concentration and thought, instead of having them interrupt me.

I use my tapes several times each day, and also every night
when I go to bed. I have condensed them onto a 120-minute cas-
sette, which gives me plenty of time to practice my relaxation
techniques and to relax enough in the evening so I can go to sleep.
One of my favorites is Dr. Siegel's tape, where you build yourself
a bridge in a corner of your own universe.[1] Another tape that is
very, very helpful to me is one pertaining to multi-hypnotic avocation.[2] In this type of tape you have two people talking about the
same subject, but in different terms. After listening to this tape,
probably 15 or 20 times, I have become able to separate the voices
and hear only the male voice or the female voice, depending upon
which one I choose to hear at that time. In the time that I am doing
this—separating the voices—it gives me great relief and great understanding of what they're saying, but it also seems to clear my

mind so that my thoughts are not as jumbled and disoriented as they are when I'm in a mood that resists relaxation.

I often have trouble concentrating in a normal day-to-day situation because my thoughts seem to run together, or they come in small pieces, like a puzzle that doesn't fit together. But, with the tapes and in a relaxed mood, I can concentrate, I can plan, and I can understand what's happening. I think this is a very fantastic field and should be utilized by everyone who has had an injury, or has been injured and is going through psychotherapy, or just as a straightforward pain-therapy program. There is a tremendous amount of material to be learned, but you must want to learn it. You cannot go to the pain-therapy session and listen to the doctor and then put the information into your dresser drawer or on your headboard and forget it. You have to use it. You must want to let this information enter your body.

You can reach a point, as I have, of being able to concentrate so deeply that you can actually see parts of your own body—you can see the injury. I have no way of proving that this is real or that it is imaginary, but to me it makes no difference. It satisfies my needs and enables me to relax and to look at my problem.

I made some mistakes in the beginning of my pain-therapy sessions. I tried to remove the injured section of my back; I tried to take the pain out and throw it away. I was very disappointed when I could not accomplish this. So, I was instructed not to try to throw it away, or make it go away, but to make friends with it, to understand it, and to ask it what its needs were, and to tell it what my needs were. This took a long time to accomplish, but I am now able to do this. At this point in my life, I still have the pain, but I understand it, I know why it's there, what its purpose is. I am not afraid of it, and even though it feels like a threat to my physical being, I know that it is not, at this time, a threat to my physical or mental well-being. When the pain reaches a challenging state, which it quite often does, I can isolate myself in some private place, and put on a tape and concentrate on it. I appear to be able, through some means I do not fully understand, to mentally release more endorphins into my body, and they go to that painful area and soothe and try to pacify the discomfort that is suffered by the injured part. I can also increase the blood flow to the area, which you can learn to do with practice. This does work. I am not a highly educated person, therefore I do not understand this, but I don't think it is completely necessary that I understand all the mechanics of it. I think it is necessary only that I believe that this will work. It will not harm me, and it will do me a tremendous amount of good, which has been proven over the last year or more.

I would like to relate one of the more fascinating experiences that I have had. And this is with the tape pertaining to taking an elevator . . . I believe this tape was made by Dr. Bernie Siegel.[3] In this exercise, you get on an elevator on the floor that represents your age. You take this elevator down and you can descend as far as you like to any year where you had a very happy experience or a very good year. You can get off and look around and examine the things that you have experienced. It is a very, very pleasant and rewarding feeling to be able to do this. There are some floors that I have been able to stop at but not able to get off at this time because of things that occurred on this floor or during this year. I can look at them from the door of the elevator, but I have not achieved the mental power or concentration to exit and walk among them. These are just things that have happened in my life—the loss of a loved one, setbacks, or like the time of my injury. I have a difficult time getting off and re-examining that. But I feel that this will be accomplished with more practice and exercise, and as I grow more mentally understanding of what I am trying to accomplish.

My thoughts are very difficult to put down, so I hope that this information can be utilized and put into a form that will assist someone else, or to help them benefit from my experiences. I sincerely believe that a person who has received an injury—and I don't think it necessarily has to be a back injury; it can be any type of trauma to your body or trauma to your psyche—should be offered the benefits of this biofeedback pain-therapy program before he/she is turned over to a surgeon.

I think the surgeon should be the last choice unless there is no choice to be made. But if options are available, I think you should go with the biofeedback/pain therapy, as far as you can, until you benefit to the point that you are able to live with your—I don't like the word "disability"—with the incapacitated portion of your body, or you can no longer tolerate the discomfort or the pain. Then you may have to go to a surgeon. The surgeons are by all means necessary, but there are numerous documented cases where people have had pain problems and have improved through the biofeed-back/pain-therapy program. This includes the use of auto-hyp-nosis, self-hypnosis, and imagery, and I have alleviated the prob-lem to the point where it no longer exists, or it exists only in a minute portion of the original condition. I don't know if medical science has any answer for this or whether you can call it a miracle. Whatever you call it, there are many things that enter into it, and this may include religion and faith. By all means, if you are a religious person, this too may help you. It may give you confidence and the ability to use your mind to help you heal yourself. The mind is a fantastic tool, and you can learn to use it in combination with your religious belief.

Surgeons are needed, but I do believe that we should try to do all that we can for ourselves before we submit to surgery. Once we submit to surgery there is no reversing that procedure. It is a removal technique, or an altering of the original design, and it cannot, in my opinion, ever be returned to its original condition.

Again, I must say that this is the most fascinating and reward-ing type of therapy that I have ever experienced. There are many books that relate to this subject, and most are in your local book-stores. There are books on biofeedback, self-healing, imagery, and other related topics. Most of the books are inexpensive, and they usually include a list of other authors who have written on a similar topic, or something that is related to the topic. These books, or at least the ones that I have had the privilege of reading, do not imply that these cures are miracles in any way. My understanding after reading some of these books is that these cures are self-procured, or self-induced healing. I think that we have a tremendous power in our minds to do these things. It is a matter of learning how to release the proper chemicals at the right time and to concentrate on the injury and/or discomfort and put it in perspective with our lives.

Some of the articles and books that I have read state that it is good to have a little pain. Pain reminds us of the probability of further damage if we are not conscious of the pain, and I do believe that this is true. If we were able to take away 100 percent of the pain and discomfort, most of us would probably go out and do some-thing that would severely damage us beyond the point of being able to live with it, or control it mentally. Then, we might have to revert to a surgical technique, but you can learn to live with a small amount of pain. It will be present most of the time in your conscious awakened state, but if you come to know it, come to make friends with it, or be on speaking terms with it, or, I should say, thinking relationship with it, it will benefit you tremendously. The discomfort is not that great as long as you can continue communicating with it. These nutrients—chemicals—come from your mind which is, I believe the most sophisticated and well-stocked pharmaceutical factory in the whole created world. It can do things and produce chemicals that I don't believe man has thought of yet.

With regard to the chemicals and such things, it has been my experience through the few medical and surgical procedures that I have had during my life span, that our whole medical experience in life is often one of using pills to cure everything. I do not wish to chastise any doctor or medical person, but I think it is just a way of life, that if you have an ache or a pain, you go to a doctor and you get a pill. I have found that it is necessary to take certain medications. I may not particularly want to, but I have to in connection with my diabetes. I have to take two injections daily to maintain my life.

We do, however, have to be very selective in what medications we take. There is a trend in this beautiful country of ours toward taking many, many medications. It has come to be my experience and my belief, since my injury, and my introduction to biofeedback, that the majority of these pain medications and tranquilizers, and whatever else is given to you can be eliminated, or very drastically cut back in their usage, if you get actively involved in the biofeedback system, and you stay with it and work with it. I don't think our bodies need all these chemicals because we can produce most of them ourselves if we take the time to understand and listen to the information that is available.

This has been a very fascinating experience for me, and I will probably continue to use it for many years to maintain the position that I now have. I am able to communicate with my inner self and with my injury and I do not take pain medication for my injury. I do take an antidepressant and an anti-anxiety medication which help me to maintain a balance with society. I think I will be able to eliminate these two drugs in the near future.

At this time, I would like to express my greatest gratitude to the doctors and psychotherapists at the treatment center. I want to give my greatest appreciation to Dr. Aleene Friedman. She is a fantastic clinician. She understands the person—she gets to know the person, and she has a tremendous way of working with you to make you feel comfortable. She has provided me with some of the most enlightening and helpful information, tapes, and procedures that have enabled me to accomplish what I have been able to do. I believe I have accomplished a great deal in the area of self-understanding and self-help, but I also believe that I am only a novice in this field of self-help, and that I have a whole world of information to learn and digest. When I accomplish this, if it can ever be completely accomplished, it will make me a much better person with regard to understanding myself, which would also allow me to understand others and to cope with my daily problems and tribulations. I hope this information will be of benefit, and I truly appreciate the opportunity to have some input into this book.

De Witt illustrates what I have often found to be a common factor in pain treatment. He states that he suffered a painful back injury and that he has chronic pain, but he goes on to elaborate on how he has suffered, over the years, from work-related emotional traumas that have caused enormous pain. This type of pain is too often discounted, especially in an environment that fosters a macho image. Until one has a visible physical injury, or has symptoms that severely interfere with one's job performance, one must, in De Witt's words, "stuff it." This causes an accumulative emotional build-up that will be vented in one's personal, social, and work life. It will also cause an additional strain on the whole organism, and may increase the likelihood of accidents and/or various types of stress-related illnesses.

De Witt demonstrates the power of imagery, and he shows how it can be utilized on a daily basis. For his part he brings to the healing partnership the ingredients that are vital to success. He brings to each session motivation and a willingness to learn that make what he has accomplished look easy. De Witt is an artist, and he is in the process of recreating and redefining his own life. He is not afraid to utilize bold strokes and brilliant colors, but neither does he avoid subtleties and muted tones that give a softness to his image. He provides us with an image of our own possibility for both pain management and change.

De Witt

My name is De Witt. I am 56 years old and I am currently being treated for chronic back pain. I have some health problems that stem from my childhood, but I am primarily dealing with the results of an industrial injury to my back and joint problems that are the result of years of wear and tear on the job. I was a fireman for over 30 years, but I am currently on a disability leave.

When I was a young fireman, I was assigned to a rescue unit. During that time one man would handle any given medical emergency call. This man, or "boot" as he was called, was usually a junior member of the fire department. Like the other young recruits I was eager to fight fires, but I could not refuse my assignment to the rescue unit. I was trained to give immediate and temporary care to the injured and/or dying. This mainly involved administering oxygen and/or bandaging wounds. I would stay with the person until an ambulance arrived, and in those days this sometimes meant a wait of 30 minutes or more. During that time I would also have to soothe the distressed family members, and sometimes I would feel helpless when a person was dying and I knew that I could not help them.

The death of a child was the most difficult rescue case to handle. Some of these calls came from parents whose child was a victim of sudden infant death syndrome (SIDS). I would sit there with a lifeless baby, listening to the resuscitator pumping oxygen into its lungs. I knew that there was no hope for the baby, but I would keep telling the parents that the baby would be alright. I didn't tell the truth and I would keep repeating "It's okay . . . it's okay, we're going to get her/him to the hospital, and everything is going to be okay." No one wanted to say, I'm sorry, your child is dead." Because of this denial of death I would sit there, time after time, with an infant growing cold and still, in my lap. We would listen to the resuscitator cycle pumping oxygen into this dead baby's lungs, until finally the ambulance would arrive, and I would return to the fire station. I went through this ordeal every time I was called on to help a dying person of any age: heart attacks, burns, drownings, accidents, or whatever it might be, it was much the same.

Regardless of how much I suffered, there was nothing to help me cope with my feelings. What I did was "stuff it." That is what everyone did. Nobody talked about a baby that had died, a burn victim's cries, or the mutilation of an accident victim. We would return to the station, and "disappear into the woodwork." Everyone would go away and deal with these things in their own fashion. In other words, we "stuffed" it. It was not "macho" to say, "Hey, that bothered me a lot." Today there are crisis intervention teams, and peer counseling is available. If these services had been available to me during my early days on the rescue unit, I might have avoided a great deal of long-term pain.

For many years I was unable to express my concerns and put them to rest. Because of my "macho" image, I learned to "stuff" it, and it was like stuffing a bag. When the bag is full, it begins to overflow. When mine began to overflow, it began to affect everything in my life: my family, my friendships, and my work. I nearly lost my family, but I used self-denial, and continued to protect my "macho" image. I would say, "There is nothing wrong with me, it's what's wrong with you," or "I'm okay, but I'm not sure about you." Finally, however, I had to admit that there was something wrong with me. I went to a mental-health specialist who served the Fire Department, and from there I was referred to a week-long workshop program called Life, Death, and Transition (LDT). During the workshop I began to express some of my feelings and to bring into the open some of my concerns, but when the week was over I did not have any after care. I did not have medication, I did not have anyone to help me to cope, and I just closed up again. I withdrew from my family and my friends because I was afraid. I was afraid to let anyone get too close to me because they, too, might die. I had held so many dying children in my arms, and I had witnessed the death of so many adults, that it seemed to me that everyone around me was in danger of dying and I could not rid myself of this fear.

My fears alienated me from my family, but they did not keep me from working. My work gave me the perfect excuse to be away from my family, and I often took extra shifts, which increased my time away from home. All of this changed, however, during a routine fire-response call. I was performing my usual duties when I noted a sharp pain in my back. I had injured myself, but, as I mentioned before, I was into being "macho" so I just went on working. The date was March 23, but I refused to fully acknowledge my injury until April 2. I finally had to admit that I could not take the pain any longer. I had a series of medical tests, and they revealed the fact that I had a ruptured disk. This is a very painful injury, but it took a lot of pain for me to admit that I needed help. I was put on the disabled list, and I will never be able to return to my job as a firefighter.

I was off from work, but I was not resolving my emotional or physical problems. I ended up seeking additional help, and I was referred to a noted psychiatrist. He immediately placed me in individual psychotherapy and individual biofeedback/pain therapy. I think that these treatment programs work best when they operate together. The psychotherapy by itself brings out a lot of problems, and lets you begin to deal with them, but it is much easier to deal with the problems and the pain if you have some additional tools to do so. My psychotherapy opened up the doors, and my biofeedback/pain therapy helped me to keep the doors open and to deal more effectively with my problems. I was fortunate in having a biofeedback therapist who was willing to participate fully in helping me to confront my problems. She had empathy, but more than that she had determination, and she wasn't afraid to confront me and to challenge me to help myself. She began to teach me some relaxation exercises, she introduced me to some very fine self-help tapes, and she provided me with home practice instructions.

There is one tape that has become my primary self-help tool.[4] This tape talks about a box and how that box can be used to contain the old images that keep coming back to haunt me. One of the things that I am dealing with is flashbacks. It is similar to what Vietnam veterans experience. I was exposed to major traumas over a period of 30 years and if I see a certain scene on the television, or in a movie, it is likely to stimulate a flashback. I have the same problem if I go into one of the areas that I worked in, or if I see an emergency situation on the road. This is beginning to improve, and I sometimes go for days at a time without thinking of the events that have so troubled me on a daily basis.

I am an accomplished artist, and my visual imagery skills are very acute. In one scene I close my eyes, and I visualize an infant who has died from sudden infant death syndrome. I am holding the infant, but then I reach out and crumple the image. It is like crumpling a photograph, and then I put this crumpled image into a box and tightly seal it inside. In the next scene I am at the seashore, and I place the tightly closed box in the water. I stand on the shoreline and watch the box float away. It becomes smaller and smaller, and eventually it goes over the horizon. At this point, it always explodes because I don't want it to ever come back. It doesn't always work, and sometimes I have to do it over and over again. Eventually it does work, and I am able to go on with what is now important to me.

There is another tape that has been absolutely invaluable to me, one that deals with decreasing my daily physical pain. This tape gets you in touch with a chemical called endorphin, which the brain secretes. This chemical is manufactured by the brain and the pituitary gland. Now I know what a brain looks like, but I don't know how it functions. I haven't the foggiest idea of what a pituitary gland looks like, nor do I have any idea what endorphins look like, but endorphins are a natural chemical pain killer that is produced by the body. They are 200 times more potent than morphine, and that really astounded me. We all know what morphine can do, but to have a chemical that is even more powerful, and produced in our body, staggers the imagination, and is almost unimaginable. I decided that I had to try to figure out a way to get these endorphins from my brain and pituitary gland to my knees and back, or wherever else I might be hurting. And I thought, well doggone it, I'm a fireman, I'll use a fire truck. So, I have imagined that there is a fire hydrant up near my brain stem that I can tap into. I can connect my fire hoses to the hydrant, and I can load the tank of my fire truck with endorphins. With my little bitsy fire truck, I can transport the endorphins to any part of my body that I need to take them to. When I heard that tape and I conceived the concept of using the fire truck to get the endorphins to the painful areas of my body, I thought, well how am I going to recognize where to put the endorphins? It came to me that the pain would be a fire, or a glowing area, and I would pull my fire truck up to that area that was painful, get off of my fire truck in my full fire-department regalia, pull my fire hoses, and apply water or endorphins to the area that was painful. Soon I could sit there with my eyes closed and watch the water being applied to the fire and feel the pain go away. I could watch it go away. This is a technique that has proven absolutely invaluable to me. I have structural injuries, and the pain keeps recurring, but I have been able to take my fire truck in there, time after time, and put the fire out. It seems to me that the intervals between recurrences of my pain are also being affected. I am going longer and longer between episodes of pain. It is a remarkable process to be able to visualize that fire truck pulling up to that emergency "hot spot" and to extinguish the pain. It really works. I may not fully understand the process, but it does work for me.

I've been asked what gets in the way of my pain control and what sets me back? What comes to the forefront are family problems. I have children, and being a relatively good parent I worry about them. I worry about what might happen to my children, and sometimes I try to help them out of difficult situations. I also have grandchildren, and stressful family situations cause increased mental and physical pain. Sometimes it is difficult to deal with some of the problems that come up, but I feel that I have the tools to help myself. At present I feel that the tapes are a great help to me. The tapes help me to relax, and almost without exception they start with taking a deep breath and slowly exhaling. That "cleansing breath" is, I feel, very important to one's recovery from disabling chronic pain. It gives you a moment to think, to back down from situations, and to attain a more relaxed state. It is a preventive pause.

As I mentioned earlier, I am an accomplished artist, and my visual imageries are vivid. Some of the imagery tapes that I like take me to a mountaintop or into colors that provide energy, or evoke a relaxation in my mind.

I have developed a place in my mind that I can go to in an instant. It is nice and warm, and there is a soft breeze. I walk across a grass-covered bank, and a small stream-fed pool glistens in the sun. There are trees that provide shade, and I can fall into that place in an instant. I feel my shoulders drop into relaxation, and I can feel the tension go out of my face. It doesn't matter where I am. I can still use this image as well as my breathing exercise. When I get angry on the road, I can go to my private imagery place and cool out, and not endanger myself or other drivers on the road. It is a safe place because I am still aware of everything around me, but I am less stressed. I use my tapes and my own visual images everyday. Sometimes while I am talking to my wife, she'll say, "I just saw you relax." I am much more responsive to my tension levels, and this has helped me to decrease my symptoms. I have learned to use what I have been taught by my biofeedback/pain therapist, and I know that others could also profit from these techniques.

I have been asked whether the therapist-patient relationship matters, and my answer to that is an unequivocal yes, it does make a difference. For example, I know people who have either bought or been given relaxation tapes. They listen to them one time, and they never get them out again because they don't understand what is being asked of them. They don't know the value of the tapes because they lack the help of a pain therapist. I think the patient needs a therapist just as a driver on a road needs the signs and markers along the road to direct them to their proper destination. Imagine trying to drive across country without any highway markers at all and you would experience the same kind of confusion that people have without the direction of a therapist. So, yes, the therapist-patient relationship is extremely important. But I think that the most important thing that you have to bring into the program is yourself. The therapist can be the best therapist in the world, but unless you, the patient, work with the therapist you cannot expect the program to be of value. It is extremely important that the patient's relationship with the therapist be nurtured.

I have included June in this pain management chapter because she is representative of the large number of people who sustain work-related injuries and receive only minimal medical care. Their chronic-pain symptoms are often ignored and tend to worsen over time. Like June, they begin to feel victimized by the system that is usually their only source of help.

The treatment costs of job-related injuries are usually excluded from one's personal health insurance policy. The patient is faced with finding a source of help that accepts a worker's compensation case and is approved for payment. Some individuals carry their own insurance policy or they are financially able to pay for their own selected treatment program. But most, like June, do not have these resources. They rely on the worker's compensation system or on lawyers who arrange for treatment on a lien basis. The system itself tends to exacerbate the patient's symptoms. It is a complex issue, but, as in June's case, one can see how difficult it is to manage pain when a partnership of healing is lacking.

June

I am a 39-year-old female. On August 5, 1988, I was injured while on my job at a local hospital. I had been working in their radiology laboratory for 2 years. I helped the patients on and off of the gurneys, and I also delivered the heavy, lead X-ray cassettes to the physicians. My work days were hectic, but I enjoyed helping the patients and working with the other members of the department.

I was injured while lifting a patient off of the gurney. I felt a sharp pain in my back and remember thinking that I must have strained a back muscle. I kept on working for several hours, but I became increasingly aware of a spreading numbness in my left arm and leg. My back, too, was becoming more painful, and finally I decided to go to the hospital emergency room. The doctor stuck a sharp needle into my left leg, and I could not feel a thing. It was obvious that I had more than a muscle injury, and the doctor ordered an MRI scan. The results of the scan showed a herniated L5 disk injury.

This injury has dramatically changed my life. For starters, my income was drastically reduced. This has been especially difficult because I am a single mother, and I have no outside support. I wanted to get back to work as soon as possible, but I had no idea how disabling the pain would be. Before my injury I was always on the go, and I exercised on a regular basis. I enjoyed an active social life and felt good about myself.

Since my accident my whole lifestyle has changed. It is difficult just to tie my shoestrings because certain movements, like bending forward, are painful. I can't exercise as actively as I once did, and I am often depressed. I tend to eat more, and I have gained weight, which adds to my distress. Sometimes I feel like I am about 80 years old.

I feel a lot more stressed than I used to because I really don't have control over important aspects of my life. It is an added stress just to deal with not knowing how I will feel from day to day, but I have also had very little treatment for my injury. I don't think that the worker's compensation system is really geared to help the patient return to their job. It seems as if the insurance companies are always fighting about how much everything costs instead of being concerned about what will benefit the patient. The doctors who have treated me were generally very impersonal. They mainly prescribed pain pills and bed rest.

I now know that it takes a long time for your body to adjust to an injury, but I also feel that much more could have been done to help me. I wanted to go to a pain clinic, but the insurance company would not approve a comprehensive treatment program. I tried to get permission to see a chiropractor or to have acupuncture treatments, but my requests were turned down. I was basically stuck with pain pills, rest, and a short-term physical therapy program. At one point I also inquired about biofeedback, but it was not available in my area. In my injury case, everyone but me has had control over my treatment program. I think that the patient should be able to express what they need to evaluate what is helping them.

It helps me to talk with people that have had the same kind of injury. They understand what I am going through and how I am feeling. It helps me to know that I am not alone, but much of the time I do feel alone in my pain. I do have some good days, but when I have added stress I have increased pain. I guess that I tighten my muscles and this causes spasms. When this happens I need to take pain pills, but my doctor wants me to stop taking pain medications. I have not taken excessive amounts of pain medications, and I feel that I will soon be left without any help for my pain.

All I want to do is to get better. I want to get my life on a normal scale as it used to be before my accident. I think that if I had known what I know now, I would have taken more control over my own situation. I would have been more demanding, and I would not have let the insurance companies push me around. A few months ago I did get a lawyer, but he is very busy and is generally unavailable.

When I was first injured, it was very difficult to live with the pain. Now, as time goes on, I've learned to deal with the pain. I have learned to live with it, and I know how to do little things that decrease my pain. I know that I can't get rid of it altogether, but I have learned some helpful techniques to alleviate the pain up to a certain point. I use breathing exercises, I pace my activities, and I listen to ocean sounds. I have learned to accept my pain, and in time you just learn to deal with it.

Marcella

This is Marcella's story, and I will tell it as best I can. There is always more to a story than can ever be told and this is especially true when the story is told by another.

Marcella was not my patient, but she had, at one time, been a chronic-pain patient. We were colleagues for five years, and she never once complained about her chronic pain. What is more, she seldom mentioned the fact that she had several other serious health problems that demanded regular health management. She was a registered nurse, but this fact had not served to protect her own health. Most of her health problems, in fact, had originated on the job.

During her last year of nursing school Marcella was assigned to work on a tuberculosis ward. At that time tuberculosis patients were kept hospitalized and isolated from their friends and family during the treatment period. The young student nurses who helped to care for these patients worked long hours and had little time for anything besides work and study. The rules for subordinates were strict, and their behavior, as well as their nursing skills, was constantly scrutinized by those who trained and supervised them. Each nursing class lived in a common dormitory area, and here, too, any infraction of the rules was cause for dismissal from nursing school.

While working on the tuberculosis ward, Marcella contracted tuberculosis and was, herself, hospitalized for a period of time. This delayed her graduation from nursing school, but once she was pronounced cured she was allowed to return and complete her nurse's training program. As I have mentioned before, there are few cures, but there are periods when disease entities are dormant. After her graduation from nursing school Marcella continued to work long hours, but she also managed to have a social life and was soon married. She often said that she knew how to take care of others, but she had never learned to take care of herself. Two years after her marriage she was diagnosed as having a recurrence of her tuberculosis, and this time major surgery was recommended. Marcella's tuberculosis-infected lung was removed and the surgical damage from this operation set the stage for a lifetime of chronic pain. The removal of her lung had forever changed the configuration of her back, and this, plus a whiplash injury, caused an added strain on the spine and other related areas.

Marcella was a young wife in her late twenties, and she wanted to have a family. Her doctors recommended that she limit herself to one child, but she ignored their advice and had what she considered the perfect family—two children. She did not, however, have the perfect husband, and she soon ended up a single mother with little outside financial support. She often talked about how hard she worked during those years and how little time she had for motherhood. She worked long hours, and she learned to dull her daily pain with the easily accessible pain medication that was made available to her. During this time she developed migraine headaches, and these too were treated with medication. She worked in a profession that believed in a pharmaceutical approach to pain, and she did not question the wisdom of ingesting large quantities of medications to control her chronic pain.

For over 20 years Marcella relied on medications to control her chronic-pain symptoms. During that time she raised her children, nursed her mother for the year prior to her death from cancer, moved from the East Coast to the West Coast, worked full time, and, in the process, developed increased pain and additional health problems. Finally Marcella sought help for herself and was treated in an outpatient pain treatment program. During this time she learned to manage her pain with a minimum of medication, and she also learned that she could contribute to the management of her migraine headaches and her hypertension. She was an excellent patient, and at the conclusion of her treatment program Marcella's biofeedback/pain therapist suggested that she consider working in the pain-management field. This was the beginning of a new career, and despite her pain, or maybe because of her own suffering, she was able to offer hope to other chronic-pain patients.

Marcella's chronic-pain patients were unaware of her own health problems, but she had a no-nonsense approach that challenged them to apply what she had so skillfully taught them. What she brought to the treatment program could only be realized in the patient/therapist relationship.

There are many "how-to" books on the market, and they provide valuable self-help tools, but healing is a gift that comes into being within the healing partnership. Marcella's pain therapist had not only guided her through the biofeedback/pain therapy program, but she had also helped her to find a meaningful way to continue to help herself and to utilize her professional skills to help others.

During the time that Marcella and I worked together we shared a sense of camaraderie. From our conversations it was apparent that her own needs, as well as the needs of others, were now being taken into consideration. The only regret that she openly expressed was that she had set an early example that made it difficult for her daughter to relax and to set aside time for herself. "It has taken me many years to know that I don't have to continually please others. I am finally able to please myself and not apologize for doing so. I can only wish the same for my daughter and my granddaughters."

The year that Marcella turned 60 she bought herself a new car. This was a life-affirming gift to herself, and we all shared her joy. Marcella continued to work until she was in her late sixties. When she entered the office, she conveyed an image that enhanced the whole environment. She had a way with color, and she often wore the lovely antique jewelry that had once been her mother's. Every person brings to a meeting with another the gift of their own self. In her early years Marcella had often depleted her own resources because her ability to give far exceeded her ability to accept something for herself. "I never felt that my own needs were important. It became more and more difficult to even acknowledge that I had needs of my own." During the last years of her life Marcella learned to love herself as well as others.

One day, while shopping for groceries, Marcella collapsed and was rushed to the hospital for emergency treatment. She underwent heart surgery and came close to dying many times during the days and weeks that followed her surgery. However, she was eventually well enough to be moved to a rehabilitation center.

I visited her at this center and realized how, in Ellen Goodman's words, medical technology does "force us to confront the paradox that the same devices that can save us can also doom us to 'a living hell.'" Marcella was secured in her wheelchair wearing a jogging suit and tennis shoes. She had thick glasses on, although it was doubtful whether she could see at all. She had feeding tubes down her throat, and had not been able to speak since her surgery. There was a need for dialysis because her kidneys were nonfunctioning, and her initial body movements seemed to be the result of uncontrolled reflex actions. I carried on a one-sided conversation, but I was not sure how much she was comprehending since her facial expression remained the same. Then I noted that she was able to make yes and no movements with her head, and I knew that she was attempting to communicate with me. As I prepared to leave her room, Marcella began to lift her right arm upward. I stood there transfixed by her slow, deliberate effort. She took over a minute to lift her hand to her face, and then she deftly brushed a tear from her eye. She slowly lowered her hand to her lap, and I quietly bade her farewell. One week later I attended her funeral.

In her editorial "Death in the Technological Age," Ellen Goodman writes:

> For much of human history, the medicine man or woman was also the caretaker. Medical mercy meant helping people, and helping people often meant helping them to die peacefully. But in our lifetime, medicine improved in its ability to save life, and doctors redefined kindness as a cure. Death becomes a technological failure . . . Our gratitude to science, our own passionate pursuit of medical salvation, now comes with increasing unease about this same technology. We fear that there may be too much of a good thing. That we can't stop it.[5]

Effective pain management is not just a matter of reducing or eliminating chronic pain. It gives one an increased ability to explore the boundaries of one's own being. When attempts to keep a person alive and/or reduce his or her pain encourage complete dependence on an outside source or a life-support system, it may be that the life that remains has little relation to living itself.

We all have our own story to tell, and it is in the telling of the story that we often find the roots of our pain and suffering, as well as the strengths that have sustained us. Life stories are seldom tales of a solitary journey. We are bound to a human existence that includes others, and the meetings and mismeetings that occur between ourselves and others have an effect upon our health and pain management.

In sharing their stories Bill, De Witt, June, and Marcella share the common factor of pain and the fact that there is no easy answer to any condition. It is in the struggle that answers are found, but these answers are never complete. They must be worked and reworked each day of our lives. I cannot abide by the simple "how-to" approach to chronic-pain management or any other aspect of life, but "how-to" steps do provide valuable tools that can be taken and personalized for one's own use. In ending this chapter I have listed some "how-to" steps that have been collected over the years from friends, relatives, and patients. Like Bill, De Witt, June, and Marcella, they are or were experts in the management of their own chronic-pain condition and/or in healing their pain.

21 Ways to Help You Manage Your Chronic Pain

1. Take a walk at least three times a week. Make this walk what I call a "focused walk." Be present in the moment and keep your thoughts from drifting to present concerns. Find what works best for you, but general simplicity facilitates a successful walking program.
2. Develop an exercise program that meets your needs. Many chronic-pain patients suffer from a state of physical deconditioning. You may need professional help to develop an appropriate exercise program, but you may also be surprised to find out how much better you feel once you are more physically fit.
3. Talk to your pain and make friends with it. Knowing your pain will help you to evaluate better what is "normal" and what is a warning signal. You will be better equipped to communicate with your own body messages and also to communicate with helping professionals.

—Lois Hulphers

4. Find ways to enjoy nature, children, and animals. Do not close yourself off from the elements of life. Keep your senses alive. Laugh, dance, and avoid being with critical people.

—Grandma Bishop (90 years old)

5. Do not feel sorry for yourself. Reach out to someone else. Take the focus off of yourself. Initiate a visit with a friend. Share a smile.

—Marian S.

6. Say no, if you need to, but do not use your pain as an excuse.

—Lil S.

7. Set your own limits. Do not let others treat you like an invalid.

—Lil S.

8. Forgive yourself and others. Go on with your life as best you can.

> —Eleanore Stephens (80 years old)

9. Use positive self-talk. Be kind to yourself. You deserve it.

> —Tilly K.

10. Dress for yourself. Wear something colorful, comb your hair, and compliment yourself.

> —Marian S.

11. Use your medications as prescribed, but begin to help yourself so that you do not become too dependent on them.

> —Jack M.

12. Live as if you have a future. Make reasonable plans for the future and create something to look forward to.

13. Get up, get dressed, and do certain basic tasks every day. It helps to have a garden or animals to tend to, but house-plants and a goldfish will suffice.

> —Grandma Allen

14. Express your feelings. If you are pleasing others at your own expense, the price is too high. Be honest and consider your own feelings.

15. Make a daily schedule. Start with the most important items and end with items that can be carried over to the next day. Be sure that you set aside time for yourself at the top of the list.

16. Use past experiences, memories of loved ones, and unfulfilled dreams to activate healing images. Each day it is important to relax and project images to yourself in a healing way.

17. Learn to adapt. Give yourself permission to change. Try doing tasks in a new way. Take breaks, get help, do a little at a time, or just do less of what has simply become an unnecessary burden. "I have to vacuum the rug every day. I like the house to look spotless." "No one can clean up the driveway and walkways as I can." Pause and evaluate how you are spending your life resources.

18. Allow for imperfections. No one is perfect, and when you strive for perfection you achieve failure. Do the best you can to help yourself and learn from what goes well and what does not.

19. Express your creativity. Creativity springs from expressing your uniqueness in the world about you.

20. Give yourself the gift of love. Love yourself and express your love to others.

21. Roll with the punches! Do not fight it, do not hang on to it, do not dwell on it. Give it your full attention when it is overwhelming. Turn your mind to other things when it is not.

—Great-grandpa Friedman

In their book *A Simple Guide for the Perplexed* (psychological first-aid), Ben Weininger and Henry Rabin try, as Ben puts it, to "hint at some ways to look at personal problems that are not usually stated simply." Ben also states:

> I have learned over many years that what changes a person's life direction from a troubled, conflicted life to a life that is more whole and meaningful is not psychology or philosophy—it is the impact made on oneself by another person. It may be a brief encounter or an enduring friendship—a relationship with a teacher or clergyman, with a stranger or with a member of our family.[6]

Ben Weininger had an impact on my life and was, I know, a great teacher/therapist to all who knew him. He and Henry Rabin have provided a simply stated comment on the complex problem of chronic pain.

When You Must Cope with Physical Pain

Pain is part of life. There are various degrees of pain and different responses to it.

For easing excessive pain, there are available chemical, meditative, hypnotic, and other remedies.

Pain and our response to it are not as simple as it seems. If there is a chronic pain, we need especially to give more consideration to its psychological components.

Pain is almost always associated with fear. A response to this pain/fear syndrome is to withdraw into ourselves. Some element of such flight usually occurs with pain.

The withdrawal is so quick that it is most difficult to observe. If we don't catch this withdrawal promptly our anxiety increases, which in turn increases our physical suffering.

Some of the more frequent fears felt by people with pain are: "I will be unable to work," "I won't be able to function," "I will not be able to cope with my social life," "I feel depressed," etc. These and many more are by-products of the withdrawal.

It is not the pain alone that is creating the withdrawal; it is also the fear of what the pain may mean. If you recognize this you will not be as restricted in your life.

There are many ways in objective reality to treat pain, but, because of the psychological withdrawal, we don't see the alternatives.

Nor do we realize that pain may be trying to give us and others a message. It may be suggesting that we re-examine our lifestyle. It may be a way of telling people close to us that we need more intimacy.

Pain is not always a negative experience. It can be a way of giving us a new direction in life.[7]

Notes

1. Bernard Siegel, "Healing meditations," Meditation Tape II, *E Cap* (Connecticut: 1988).
2. "Rapid Pain Control Tape," *The Changeworks* (Berkeley).
3. Bernard Siegel, "Healing meditations," Meditation Tape I, *E Cap* (Connecticut: 1988).
4. Emmett Miller, "Accepting change—Moving on," *Tape Source* (Stanford: 1981).
5. Ellen Goodman, "Death in the technological age," *Los Angeles Times* (December 28, 1990, editorial page).
6. Ben Weininger and Henry Rabin, *A Simple Guide for the Perplexed: Psychological First-Aid* (Van Nuys: Creative Book, 1987), p. 7.
7. Ibid., p. 40.

CHAPTER 16

Chronic Acute Pain

Most of us can remember a time of acute pain, but we also remember that it was a temporary condition. Medications, medical or dental interventions, or time itself may have helped to diminish the pain. When a painful condition becomes a chronic condition, it disrupts one's life. But when chronic pain escalates to a chronic acute stage it further removes the person from all but their own painful existence. It is a very lonely, subjective experience. It is difficult for others to fully acknowledge another person's pain. Each person needs to maintain his or her own ground, and another person's suffering may threaten his or her own sense of security in the world. This may be one reason why we so often isolate the aged, ill, and dying in our society. We do not like to come face to face with our own mortality, and pain is often associated with the loss of life.

We do not have an exact scientific measurement device to determine the demarcation line between chronic pain and chronic acute pain. There are, however, certain chronic conditions that are recognized as disorders that generate acute pain. These conditions include trigeminal neuralgia, advanced stages of cancer, and severe arthritis. If patients themselves were asked about their chronic-pain levels, I'm sure that those with debilitating back pain, frequent severe migraine headaches, and assorted other conditions might well emphasize the severity of their own chronic pain.

Whatever the level of pain, the issue of pain management must be addressed. I think that all patients would agree that increased chronic-pain symptoms intensify the patient's need for pain management. This becomes an especially difficult task if pain medications have been the primary method of control. In time the patient's tolerance of pain medications increases and there is a "rebounding effect" that causes increased pain as the medication effect "wears off." This may begin to occur on a more frequent basis, and the solution is seldom one of increased dosages. The patient, however, may become extremely demanding and angry when medication is withheld and/or closely monitored.

Some of the most effective pain-relief medications are highly addictive and often produce a condition of stupor. When to start administering these medications to the terminally ill is an ongoing issue. I have occasionally been asked to help a terminally ill cancer patient manage his/her chronic acute pain. This request tends to come at a time when the patient's pain symptoms are rapidly elevating, but the disease, itself, is not yet at a crisis stage. Thus, the patient may be denied the more potent medications that are reserved for the last stages of the disease.

I highly recommend that pain therapy sessions be started early in the treatment program, and that they be included in a comprehensive multidimensional treatment program that emphasizes healing, wellness, and pain management. As a person's pain level increases, his/her ability to integrate new material decreases. In his article "The World of the Patient in Severe Pain of Long Duration," Lawrence Le Shan provides an in-depth study of the effects of long-term chronic acute pain and also suggests ways to augment therapeutic interventions within the patient's treatment program.

> If we observe the world with which we are concerned here— the *universe* of the patient in chronic pain—we can perceive a similarity to the universe of the nightmare. If we look at the terror dream, and ask what are its structural components, we see that there are three basic ones: (1) terrible things are being done to the person and worse are threatened; (2) others, or outside forces, are

in control and the will is helpless; (3) there is no time-limit set, one cannot predict when it will be over. The person in pain is in the same formal situation: terrible things are being done to him and he does not know if worse will happen; he has no control and is helpless to take effective action; no time-limit is given. This aspect of the psychic assault upon the integrity of the ego that accompanies severe, chronic pain is a major one: the patient lives during the waking state in the cosmos of the nightmare.

This is further emphasized by the meaninglessness and inexplicability of pain. Mental suffering seems to follow naturally from our thoughts and actions: with the possible exception of some of the obsessive compulsive states, it is somehow organic to us, syntonic to our views of ourself. Chronic pain is alien; it seems to indicate an utter senselessness. It appears to be meaningless and so, since it is very hard for man to accept that real experience may be unreasonable, we attempt to give it meaning. Our ancient guilts and anxieties are aroused, and we try to assign our pain to these insufficient causes. Although this is a frequent reaction, it rarely leads, for individuals of our society, to a useful sense of meaning.

The meaning of pain has been approached by every great religion and philosophy. In our own anti-metaphysical culture it is largely ignored. This lack of a perceived meaning, of a culturally understood context, makes it much harder for the individual to deal with chronic pain. As the Nazis well understood and demonstrated, meaningless and purposeless torture is much harder for the person to accept and resist than is torture which the subject can place in a coherent frame of reference. A perceived senselessness in the universe weakens our belief that our efforts have validity and point. They appear to be essentially futile. This makes it much harder to continue these efforts, including those of coping with pain and stress.

It is common, in our generalization from acute to chronic pain, to assign to pain the idea of a warning; a signal that something is wrong and that we should do something about it. This orientation often makes it more difficult for the therapist to be clear about the problems involved. Scheler points out that the sensation of weariness says "rest," dizziness at the edge of an abyss says "step back," and hunger that one should eat. Chronic pain, however, indicates only a state of existence. It does not warn or tell us what to do. It does not help us act and may be so severe as to disrupt potentially useful activities and habits. The adequate expression of thirst is to drink. The adequate expression of this kind of pain is only a scream.

Another aspect of the psychic assault made by severe pain is implied in this. It is related to the fact that it is important to ourselves that we respond to strong stimuli; that we are connected to and react to the environment. With pain this is much more difficult; we are constantly pushed towards suffering rather than interacting. We cannot act, we can only bear. Time and space are the basic framework for our exchanging energy with the cosmos and thus replenishing the strength of our psychic coherence. Pain weakens our relationship with this framework. There is a pulling to the center, a centripetal force that brings our energies and our consciousness into ourselves and away from all else and all others. When he has no real goals in time, the inner life decays. There is a real loss of time perspective in pain—we are pulled in the immediate. The intensity and duration of the stimulus binds us to it. Our libidinal energy is pulled back from its objects and used as a defensive wall against the pain. However this shift of the libido increases our focusing of attention on the pain and thereby makes it fill our life-space to a greater degree and reduces our ability to deal with it. The lost objects can no longer sustain us and help us maintain our inner integrity and sense of being, purpose and meaning. Pain permits personal existence to continue with little assistance from our usual orientations, defenses, safeguards and associations. It attenuates our relationships with the outer world at the same time that it weakens the inner structure. In painless consciousness we are filled with images, associations, thoughts. In the loud loneliness of pain, only our existence is real. We float alone in space, conscious only of the suffering.

These reactions and the passive, helpless quality of being in chronic pain tend to press us strongly towards a psychic regression. Our dignity and our hard-won adult status is weakened. The body image—our sense of our physical aspects and a basis of our sense of being, our *persona*—is blurred as the pain seems to obliterate the rest of the body. We are conscious only of the area that is providing the overwhelming sensations. The ego strength is further weakened by this reduction of complexity of the organization of the adult perception of the body. It returns us to the body-image (and, with this, the feelings, the helplessness and dependency) of childhood. This is further added to by the fact that when we are in severe pain we, as in childhood, have to depend on others to take the important actions in our lives.

This is one reason that pity for the person in pain is an extremely corrosive emotion and—when perceived by the patient—further makes less his ability to deal with the situation. The pity reinforces the regression through its implication of a lower status. The strivings to retain dignity and adulthood can be reinforced through empathy, emotional contact and respect. Pity only weakens them . . . The emotional state, the "*lebensegefühl*," determines in large part the perception of pain, and its power over a person. One woman who had had terribly severe pain for many years from an inner ear disorder, but who had continued her active, useful and ebullient life in spite of this, responded to the question of how she did it by saying, "When the pain is severe, I rise above it and look at it from a higher level." To dismiss this remark and technique as 'hysteroid' would be missing the entire point. She retained command over herself and the pain and so was not overwhelmed as a person by it. Her psychic structure remained intact and master of her fate.[1]

Le Shan has discussed the general situation of "the person in pain." "It may," he states, "be worthwhile also to be aware of some specific aspects which may play a part in the total situation." He goes on to say:

> These special aspects are possibilities that it appears advisable to keep in mind before action against the pain is taken by means of drugs, suggestions, hypnosis or other methods.

When the patient and the therapist enter into a healing partnership the patient has the opportunity to communicate the underlying aspects of his or her pain. This is more likely to happen when the therapist actually listens to the patient and does not try to listen for the underlying aspects of the patient's pain. Many chronic-pain patients avoid psychotherapy because they do not like having their pain symptoms psychologized. The specific aspects that Le Shan is referring to are:

1. Pain as communication. Here, he utilizes Szasz's writings to illustrate how a person's pain may be his or her main way to communicate a need for help. "It can be a way of stating a psychic situation."
2. Pain as an answer to psychic needs. Le Shan recapitulates how "Engel, Cangello and others have discussed in some detail the use of pain to fill an inner need: to maintain the psychodynamic structure of the person."[2]

There is, I feel, a danger of not fully listening to the patient if one is searching for the underlying aspects of the patient's pain condition. I do agree, however, that time should be given to explore these possibilities, but I strongly feel that this is best accomplished in a program that is enhanced by a moderate level of medication intervention, self-help programs such as biofeedback pain therapy, and other programs that are appropriate for the individual needs of the patient suffering from chronic pain. When this is lacking there is more likelihood that the pain may elevate to a chronic acute state of pain. I think that this may also be true for the person who is suffering from cancer. There is too much focus on invasive treatments and too little focus on how the patient can help himself/herself. The fear of pain is an important factor in cancer, and it is much more difficult to help a patient who has reached chronic acute pain. What does seem to help is short sessions that focus on quiet breathing and other calming exercises. Ocean waves or healing music are also helpful. The patients' tolerance for input needs to be taken into consideration and respected.

Le Shan's sensitivity and insights, in relation to the care of patients with chronic acute pain, adds important dimensions and implications that are relevant for both the therapist and the patient.

Some Guidelines for the Therapist

The hardest task for the therapist, and yet perhaps the most basic, is to help the patient arrive at a meaning, at making some sense out of what is happening to him. Here, there can be no rules as to how this is done, only an orientation as to its importance. Each patient must be helped to the path most syntonic to *him*, to his own sense of meaning, not the meaning that makes sense to the therapist. His uniqueness is crucial and the knowledge of this, in itself, may be helpful. To know—to be reinforced in the knowledge—that one is unique and irreplaceable—as a loved one or one who loves, as one with special tasks, or in some other manner—gives much support to the psychic structure and the ability to handle the situation. (This is one reason why experiments with pain-relieving agents often have such positive effects on the control subjects who are receiving only placebos. Their participation in the experiment itself reinforces their status as individual persons, increases their ability to deal with the pain and thus decreases their perception of it.) One patient was able to understand the connection between her pain and the healing process; that the pain was an inexorable part of treatment. She said, "Now that I know there is a reason, I feel it much less and can keep doing things when it comes. It's like the difference between childbirth and the other pains. In labor you know something will be produced at the end. It's never as bad as when the pain doesn't produce anything."

It is perhaps important for the therapist first to be clear about his own feelings in this area before he can effectively help the sufferer. If he believes that there *is* a meaning, even if he cannot find it, he is in a much better position to help . . .

One patient who had suffered very severe pain for a long period, and still was in acute, physical distress, said, "Sometimes with a lot of pain, a person becomes *verklärt* (clarified) and all the trivial, unimportant things become unimportant. You stop spending your life worrying about them."

Other patients can understand that the experience they have had can never be taken from them, that after it is over they will never need to fear anything again and that, as Nietzsche put it, "That which does not kill me, makes me stronger." Other patients may see the pain they have as *existing in itself* and *their* experiencing it saves someone else from the experience. Each patient must be helped to his own solution. The effectiveness of the psychotherapist depends, in large part, on his ingenuity in helping the patient to the best answer for him as an individual. It is the knowledge of the importance of this that is central for the therapist. Dostoevski said, "There is only one thing I dread, not to be worthy of my sufferings." In this dark and wise sentence we see the need for the emergence and maintenance of the self in the welter of pain.

A second major guideline for the therapist is to help the patient find ways to act and react to the situation: to help the patient take some semblance of control over his situation. In the act of control, much strength is given to the inner being: the person is strengthened. Sometimes the patient must be helped to understand that for certain tasks, the action that is called for is to do nothing but to wait and bear and that this can be an active, not a passive, process. This can be a very valuable insight to some patients.

Frequently the patient feels he can only "be brave and heroic" or surrender. This can be an impasse which demands more than the patient has to give. The value of "a stiff upper lip" is often vastly overestimated by both the patient and those around him. Sometimes just permission to cry ("some things are worth a few tears") reduces the rigidity and makes it possible for other responses to take place. This should not be done, however, with the patient with a rigid, brittle ego which may be overwhelmed and drowned by a passive-dependent flood. In these patients it is necessary rather to reinforce [sic] the rigid defenses (often with obsessive-compulsive techniques) than to weaken them.

One can also help some patients to understand the concept that the facts, including the facts of our inner life, are not as important as our attitude toward them. In the old story where one soldier was reproached and ridiculed by another for feeling fear under shellfire, the first answered: "It shows we are different, but it does not show I am inferior. If you were one-half as frightened as I am, you would have run away long ago." The "fact" of pain impulses is also less important to the person's ability to deal with them than his attitude toward them.

A third lead for the therapist sometimes may be to make the "nightmare" conditions conscious. To understand clearly the psychic pressures on a person, sometimes make them much easier to resist. Not only do we understand that the pressures and our re-actions are "natural," "expected," but also that they are universal and not special and secret to us. Further, the more an emotion and its causes are looked at clearly and objectively, the weaker it tends to become.

One major way of helping the patient in pain is to help him remove the focus of concentration from the pain to outside events. The pain is felt to be worse when it occupies the entire life field. Work, occupational therapy, relating to others: these things do much more than just "pass the time." They also diminish the pain. Both "attention" and "consciousness" are essential to the perception of pain. We can reduce one or the other, but the reduction of "attention" can often be surprisingly effective.

In the demand the psychotherapist makes that the patient turns his energies outward from the pain and that he function as a person, the therapist should avoid being too "soft" and gentle. He can make high demands; this indicates far more respect and consequently strengthens the person far more than overconcern. The same orientation that we have toward mental anguish in psychotherapy is called for here. To be loving and demanding is a difficult road to walk, but it is the road that gives the greatest support and help to the patient. Sometimes the therapist can be aided in this if he asks himself whether his goal for the patient is painlessness or if it is composure, dignity and mastery.

Each of us lives in a unique, existential universe. The effectiveness of the psychotherapist who would relieve suffering is related to his understanding of, and empathy with, the universe of the sufferer. This is as true for the person with severe chronic pain as it is for those whose anguish is felt in the emotional sphere. It is also true, however, that the universes of those in pain tend to have common trends and pressures which appear to have implications for the therapist. This paper has been an attempt to describe some of these commonalities.[3]

Sophie

Sophie's trigeminal neuralgia had been a source of chronic acute pain for over a year. Her symptoms were the center of her life and a major source of all that went on between her husband and herself. Sophie and her husband, Alex, were introduced to me a day or so before her first appointment. She had been hesitant about entering a biofeedback/pain therapy program, and a staff nurse was trying to assure her that this was an appropriate program for her. She looked skeptical, and I also tried to assail her doubts. Sophie looked me in the eye and stated: "Every person that I have seen has felt that they could help me, but they haven't. This pain is going to kill me, and that will probably be the only thing that will actually stop the pain. We will be here for my appointment, but I hope that it is not a waste of our time and money." I cannot say that I was looking forward to our appointment, but I had learned that many patients, who are initially what would be called difficult patients, actually do quite well.

Some patients are more difficult to treat than others, and this is especially true of patients with chronic acute pain. Some may have unreasonable expectations, but others, like Sophie, live with little or no hope that their pain will diminish. There is usually a history of previous treatment programs that have failed to produce satisfactory results, and this is bound to have at least an initial impact on their current treatment program. When you are in pain you have an urgent need for results, and this is a factor that often impedes the results that are so desperately sought after.

Sophie was exactly on time for her appointment, and she was accompanied by her husband. During this initial session I tried to lay the groundwork that would make it clear that this type of treatment program involved an element of shared responsibility. I would serve as her teacher/therapist, and my responsibility was to guide and support her while helping her to help herself. She would need to utilize home practice instructions and incorporate what she learned into her everyday life. Sophie's discomfort was obvious, but she was verbal and articulate throughout the session.

The sensitivity of Sophie's mid-body areas and parts of her upper back caused, in her words, excruciating pain. It was difficult for her to sit comfortably, and anything that touched the affected areas caused increased pain. This meant that showering and/or bathing caused pain and that lying down or sitting up had to be done with great care. Just the touch of her clothing was a source of pain. Heat and/or cold could not be used to comfort her, but a warm room was more desirable. Even a gentle flow of air that circulated around her body could provoke a painful response.

Sophie estimated that her pain level fluctuated between five and ten on a scale of one to ten. Five was considered moderately severe and ten was rated as excruciating. She had periods of relief while sleeping, but she seldom slept for more than 3 hours at a time. As I was to find out later, music was her one great solace, but she was at this time unwilling to share this fact.

Alex was the family record keeper. He had carefully recorded the dates and costs of Sophie's previous treatment modalities. The list was long and represented a sizable expense. Alex made it clear that he would check on their insurance coverage before scheduling a series of pain-therapy sessions. They were living on a budget, and it was obvious that every expenditure was accounted for. As it turned out, they did have adequate medical coverage for the pain-therapy sessions, and he cautiously scheduled a series of five sessions. This was, in my opinion, the minimum number of sessions needed to ascertain whether Sophie was benefiting from the program.

Sophie and Alex were a team, and it was necessary to work with both of them. Sophie did much of the talking, but Alex filled in the gaps and was quick to verify the truth of Sophie's statements. They had been married over 40 years and both were intelligent, well-read, and highly critical of anything or anyone who failed to meet their high standards. Alex's list was long and went beyond the medical interventions and the various health professionals who had failed to produce satisfactory results.

The first introductory session of biofeedback/pain therapy is, in a sense, a pivotal session. Patients leave the program at various points, but during this first session the decision to return and make at least a minimal commitment is determined. The patient does not walk out of this session with a clear picture of what is to be accomplished, but he or she does gain a sense that there is some hope of effecting a positive change in their condition. Alex and Sophie managed to control effectively most of the various aspects of their personal life, but Sophie's illness was out of control. I knew that it was important to help them to gain a sense of control over this aspect of their lives.

I introduced Sophie to the use of an electromyograph (EMG) to measure selected muscle-tension levels. These levels were monitored with sensors that were placed over various upper-body sites. It was important to select areas that were not sensitive to touch, but might be exacerbating her symptoms. First, I chose to monitor the facial area and later added the upper-shoulder area. It was easy to see that Sophie's frustration and pain had caused tightness in the facial muscles, and in this area there was little danger of aggravating her mid-body pain.

Many patients do not want a detailed, step-by-step explanation of their treatment program, but I was sure that attention to detail would be important to Sophie and Alex. I explained how tension in one area of the body may cause increased tension in another part of the body, or conversely how relaxing one area of the body may serve to send a calming message throughout the nervous system. I was monitoring the facial muscles at rest. Like her pain level, the tension levels over the frontalis (forehead) were very high. They ranged from eight to ten on a scale of one to ten. Even with the eyes closed the EMG levels of tension were high, but when she was shown how to relax the masseter muscles (jaw muscles), there was a significant reduction in her levels of tension. Relaxing the lower facial area can be combined with a simple breathing exercise, and this same breathing exercise can eventually be expanded to attain the deeper sense of calming that comes when we reduce high levels of tension throughout our body. This was another lesson, and, for now, Sophie was given home practice instructions and a facial relaxation tape. We set some goals and a time for her second session of pain therapy.

In many ways Alex and Sophie were living a nightmare existence, but a large part of their nightmare seemed to be connected to their dislike of being dependent on others who seemed incapable of helping them. The more credentials a health professional had the more caustic their comments were. (They were very proud people, and they would not have allowed anyone's pity to damage their sense of dignity.) I focused on what Sophie could do for herself and during each session she could visually see that it was possible to decrease her muscle-tension levels. This, of course, needed to be paired with some decrease in the symptoms, but both Sophie and Alex liked to see that the initial tension levels were slowly dropping. I explained that it takes time to re-educate the body to let go of chronic tension and that for lasting results one needs to generalize the skills into the patterns of everyday living. They understood this and did not feel frustrated by the lack of a significant drop in Sophie's pain level.

I was still looking for what it was that had helped Sophie to handle past stressors. During our third session together she informed me that she had once been an accomplished pianist. "I loved playing the piano and I would often practice for hours at a time. Now I find sitting on the piano bench causes too much discomfort, and my playing no longer meets my own high standards." What Sophie currently loved was listening to the local classical music radio station. I suggested that she spend some time imagining herself playing the piano, especially while she was listening to a favorite piece of music. While she was doing this, I wanted her to see herself as relaxed and doing well.

I utilize the various biofeedback modalities to help each patient gain a better understanding of how he/she can begin to help himself/herself. The audio and visual signals provide instant feedback, but this type of feedback should become less necessary in time. The goal is to bridge the communication gap that has existed within the person's sphere of being without creating a dependence on the biofeedback equipment.

When Alex suggested buying a portable EMG unit for Sophie to practice with at home, I did not encourage him to do so, but it soon became apparent that both Alex and Sophie were determined to follow through on this plan. I provided them with my file on EMG biofeedback units, and Alex was soon at work researching each of the various models.

Sophie had one session left, and we continued to focus on various ways to divert her attention from her symptoms. She had less pain while she was concentrating on the biofeedback signals, and she had decreased the levels of tension over the facial and shoulder areas. She was now working on generalizing these specific tension-reduction skills to the rest of the upper-body areas. Sophie felt that just eliminating the weekly ride to my office was going to help her. Quick stops, bumpy roads, and any jarring movements increased her symptoms. She dreaded all but the shortest of trips in the car. Now she would be able to practice everyday, and she would not have to endure the 30-minute ride to my office.

Two weeks later Alex called to tell me about the arrival of the EMG unit. He was very pleased that the unit was working well, and we set up a time for me to meet with him and Sophie during the next week. Being with Sophie, in her home environment, revealed how the complexity of her pain was bound up in the patterns of her everyday life. They lived in a quiet, lovely neighborhood, but they had, in every possible way, shut themselves off from the outer environment. They lived behind closed, barred windows, iron-gated screen doors, and security-locked exterior doors. The rooms lacked fresh air and no other forms of life dwelt here. A grand piano dominated the living room and books spilled out from every nook, shelf, and cranny in the room. Sophie was reclined on the couch and had the EMG unit set up in front of her. She demonstrated how well she was doing, and indeed her readings were moderately low. She stated that she had not yet approached the piano, but felt that she would do so if she continued to improve. Alex busied himself with the stack of paperwork on his desk but occasionally joined in during the flow of conversation. They both seemed relaxed, and they were surrounded by memories of the past.

Many photographs of friends and former colleagues were framed and displayed around the room. Sophie named each of these people and explained his or her relationship to Sophie and Alex. Some of the people had been writers and others scientists, and all had been a part of their social circle. The photographs were at least 40 years old, and all the subjects were deceased. It appeared that Sophie and Alex had been young protegés of at least some of the members of this group. She showed me their former summer home on the East Coast, which had served as a gathering place for their many friends. It was a large, inviting house, and guests were assembled on the front porch for a group picture. The gap between their former socially active life and their present closed-off life was a mystery, but according to Sophie they had never met new friends that could measure up to their old ones. It appeared that as the old life had died away they had clung to their memories and each other. Sophie had told me that they had decided not to have children because they felt that the future was too uncertain. It was during this conversation that Sophie told me that I could have been her daughter.

Alex and Sophie were sometimes lonely and frightened, but they were not devoid of a rich, inner world. They read and discussed books, loved music, kept up with the news, and occasionally went to lectures. There was a demand for detail and a lack of flexibility that created some of Sophie's chronic tension. They were both critical and perfectionistic, and this, too, contributed to Sophie's pain. Yet her sense of control over the pain had improved. I felt that I had helped Sophie to handle her pain more effectively, but I knew that I could not assuage the painful knowledge that she had severed her connection to the future. She was in danger of facing the future alone, and she clung desperately to the past. I could not become the daughter that Sophie now wished for, and it was time to leave because I had reached the limit of my own resources. I was pleased that Sophie had improved, and our farewell wishes were warm and caring. I knew that being able to say goodbye to Alex and Sophie did not mean that I would be able to forget them.

Notes

1. Lawrence Le Shan, "The world of the patient in severe pain of long duration," *Journal of Chronic Disease,* Vol. 17 (1969), pp. 119–122.
2. Ibid., p. 122.
3. Ibid., pp. 123–125.

CHAPTER 17

Preventing Chronic Pain

I have mentioned in an earlier chapter that while much has been written on the benefits of preventive health care, it is still the dramatic effects of advanced technology that support most of our large health-care treatment centers. Many people seek to replace and/or restore worn-out parts of their body, and there is the hope of regaining one's health when the effects of extreme wear and tear have diminished the quality of one's life.

Much of the material on preventive health care is incorporated within the numerous "how-to" books. These books are usually directed at a population that has health problems but wants to prevent the serious consequences that might occur if the problems are not addressed. Subjects for "how-to" books include: improving fitness levels, regulating blood pressure, curing headaches, improving sleep, controlling chronic pain, and losing weight. There are, of course, articles and books that actually do feature healthy lifestyles and preventive health care, but the impact of this material may not be as widespread because pain and discomfort are primary movers.

Joan Borysenko's book *Minding the Body, Mending the Mind* is an excellent example of a "how-to-help-yourself" book. The cover description of this book states:

Joan Borysenko has created the first systematic medically tested

program to unlock the mind's power to manipulate health . . .
Patients come to the Mind/Body Clinic with ulcers, migraine, gastritis, and they come with cancer and heart disease.[1]

The daily periods of meditation and the other aspects of the Mind/Body Clinic are very beneficial for the patients. What we also need are other basic programs, like this one, that work to prevent the chronic problems that these patients suffer from. There is too much emphasis on human repair and not enough on preventive care. Borysenko emphasizes the art of self-repair, despite the fact that she is clearly an important part of this health-care program. It is obvious that she often forms a healing partnership with her patients and that there are healing benefits for both the patients and Borysenko.

Because preventive health care is not a primary focus in our society, the need for healing is reaching epidemic proportions. Healing is needed throughout our society, but the prevention of chronic disorders and/or chronic pain is equally basic and can only happen through loving, nurturing, and protecting our children. The way we cope with physical and emotional injuries, the availability of resources when we are confronted with pain, our ways of expressing pain, and the pain that we carry within us are directly related to our earliest experiences of emotional and/or physical pain.

Only during the last 5 years has the medical world officially acknowledged that infants experience pain. This has influenced pediatric surgical procedures and possibly aided those who expressed concern about childbirth procedures. Many babies in our country suffer because their needs are not being met before or after their births. At least 40,000 of these babies die every year, and many others will develop chronic disorders.

The rhythms of life pulsate in and around the developing embryo and continue to do so throughout the fetus's full cycle of development. The comforting sounds of the mother's heartbeat, the flow of her blood as it circulates throughout the body, and the other sounds of this interior world become at one with the fetus. He/she picks up the rhythm and expresses the emotional/physical state of the mother within his/her own body. Under the best of circumstances the fetus dwells in a protective environment that nurtures the growth and development that are necessary for life outside of the womb.

For some, the rhythms of stress and possibly pain are introduced by a daily bombardment of life-threatening agents and the distress signals of a troubled mother. The nutrients for growth and development may be lacking, and survival becomes an issue. The life rhythms that are developed in the womb of these mothers are not those that promote health and well being. Once these babies are born, they are usually less lovable and more difficult to care for. This may also apply to premature babies who are thrust into the world before they are physically able to sustain life on their own. Westley was a premature twin who did not thrive as well as his brother. His brother was more responsive and lovable and this created a serious problem for his mother, D. Merlin, and for Westley. The following quote is excerpted from the *Los Angeles Times.*

> Westley came home at four months, weighing just seven and one half pounds. He was so weak, it would take hours to feed him two ounces of milk. He seemed withdrawn, in pain and physically rigid. He would sit in his swing, sucking on a pacifier and avoiding eye contact . . . "When I went to hold Westley he would cry . . . " After Westley's fourth rehospitalization, the Merlins hired a nurse who specialized in high-risk infant care. She began working with Westley—exercising his limbs, giving him physical therapy and distracting and comforting him when he cried in pain. Within ten days, Merlin recalls, Westley was crying to be held. "It changed my relationship with him," said Merlin. "I think about what could have happened if the nurse hadn't taken over the case . . . " "Westley was definitely developing a behavior problem because he wasn't bonding with me, with people." "He was developing social problems, social retardation. Then he came out of his shell. People are drawn to him now."[2]

Merlin and others believe that many parents, physicians, and health officials fail to recognize the importance of early medical, educational, and family support in maximizing the potential—and improving the lives—of babies born underweight.

Westley's nurse formed a healing partnership with him and in so doing called him into being. Every child needs the confirmation of personal address and the gentle expressions of love that are first communicated on a sensate level.

When children are made to endure emotional deprivation and/or physical abuse over a prolonged period of time, the tortured child may eventually become the torturer. It has been estimated that over 80% of America's prison population, 90% of all first-degree murderers, and almost 100% of child abusers were abused children.

The cycle of abuse that moves from one generation to another is also related to the underlying causes of chronic pain and/or chronic conditions. One has only to listen to patients to know the truth of this statement.

We are a society that goes to great lengths to keep a dying infant alive, but maintains a collective silence when that same child dies a slow death from the ravages of poverty, neglect, and physical and/or mental abuse. Many children of all ages are imprisoned in a nightmare world that does not call them into being. They exist, but they are denied the opportunity to develop a sense of self, and this is the basic denial of their right to be in the world.

In her book *The Body in Pain: The Making and Unmaking of the World*, Elaine Scarry addresses the issue of torture. The elements of torture that she so skillfully outlines and discusses in her book are relevant to the situation of many infants and children who become prisoners of "torture" in their own homes. The memories of this torture, or abuse, may remain well hidden, but what the memory fails to reveal will be released within the body. Each new injury and/or illness will add new insults to an already damaged structure, and in time the resources to sustain pain may diminish as will the will to live.

Scarry offers us an intricate analysis of the elements of torture, but, for the purposes of this book, I have selected only a limited number of passages which are, I feel, basic to the issue at hand.

The first area discussed is what Scarry refers to as the "unmaking of the world."

> It is the intense pain that destroys a person's self and world, a destruction experienced spatially as either the contraction of the universe down to the immediate vicinity of the body or as the body swelling to fill the entire universe. Intense pain is also language-destroying: as the content of one's world disintegrates, so the content of one's language disintegrates; as the self disintegrates, so that which would express and project the self is robbed of its source and its subject.
>
> Torture . . . consists of a primary physical act, the infliction of pain, and a primary verbal act, the interrogation. The verbal act, in turn, consists of two parts, "the question" and "the answer," each with conventional connotations that wholly falsify it. "The question" is mistakenly understood to be "the motive"; "the answer" is mistakenly understood to be "the betrayal." The first mistake credits the torturer, providing him with a justification, his cruelty with an explanation. The second discredits the prisoner, making him rather than the torturer, his voice rather than his pain, the cause of his loss of self and world.[3]

The four aspects of pain that Scarry so succinctly outlines further serve to illustrate the elements of pain and torture.

> —The first, the most essential, aspect of pain is its sheer aversiveness. While other sensations have content that may be positive, neutral, or negative, the very content of pain is itself negation. If to the person in pain it does not feel averse, and if it does not in turn elicit in that person aversive feelings toward it, it is not in either philosophical discussions or psychological definitions of it called pain . . .
>
> —A second and third aspect of pain, closely related to the first, are the double experience of agency. While pain is in part a profound sensory rendering of "against," it is also a rendering of the "something" that is against, a something at once internal and external. Even when there is an actual weapon present, the sufferer may be dominated by a sense of internal agency: it has often been observed that when a knife or a nail or pin enters the body, one feels not the knife, nail or pin but one's own body, one's own body

hurting one. Conversely, in the utter absence of any actual external cause, there often arises a vivid sense of external agency, a sense apparent in our elementary, everyday vocabulary for pain: knife-like pains, stabbing, boring, searing pains. In physical pain, then, suicide and murder converge, for one feels acted upon, annihilated by inside and outside alike . . .

—This dissolution of the boundary between inside and outside gives rise to a fourth aspect of the felt experience of physical pain, an almost obscene conflation of private and public. It brings with it all the solitude of absolute privacy with none of its safety, all the self-exposure of the utterly public with none of its possibility for camaraderie or shared experience.[4]

Elaine Scarry's work is aimed at the global aspects of torture within the political/social forces of the world. Her writings, however, also challenge us to address the politics of the family and the social forces that facilitate the maiming, murder, and continued neglect of large numbers of children within our culture. There is a silence that protects the politics of the family while denying the legitimate right of the child to exist fully. This goes beyond "unmaking the world," because the child is denied a world of his/her own, from the outset of life.

Four years ago I was invited to a bris, the Jewish ritual of circumcising a male child when he is 8 days old. It was to be a day of celebration, but the rabbi who performed the circumcision created an atmosphere of pain and apprehension. The slow, meticulous movements of his scissors caused the baby to convulse with pain. Eventually, his sister began to fear for her brother's life and had to be removed from the room and reassured that he was not in mortal danger.

The social/religious structure of this ritual event did not allow for an adult protest. The baby was restrained, and the adult community sat in silence. This baby was subjected to an unusually painful circumcision, but most of his young life would be one of protection and love. He was surrounded by family members who would provide loving care and it was likely that this would help him to heal. Not every child is as fortunate as this child.

Stephen

Stephen was tortured throughout his infancy and childhood, but his is not a worst-case scenario. His bones were not broken, he was not visibly brain-damaged, and he was not killed by his torturer. Stephen was also spared the torture of prolonged periods of isolation and/or severe neglect. What did add to his suffering was the conspiracy of silence that protected his abusive father, for it denied his pain.

Stephen's middle-class parents had initially welcomed him into the world. He was a handsome, healthy baby, and members of the extended family had also been delighted by his birth. During his first 3 months of life Stephen began to emerge from his drowsy newborn state, and he was increasingly more vocal about his own needs. His father soon decided that it was time to curb the incessant demands of this little "tyrant." From that moment Stephen was seldom fed or tended to "on demand." His parents took care of his needs when it was convenient for them to do so. The first element of torture is pain, and Stephen's father, an abused child himself, began to inflict pain on a regular basis. The second element is the interrogation. In Stephen's case, there was often an indirect interrogation, followed by a direct interrogation. Stephen's mother would be asked: "What's wrong with the little brat?" She would answer: "I don't know, maybe he is hungry again. I'll get to him in a few minutes." Stephen's cries would soon permeate the whole house, and then he would be interrogated: "What makes you think that your needs are the only ones that count in this household?" "Who do you think you are?" "Do you know that you are a tyrant?" The "question and answer" period was a formality that emphasized the child's guilt. The questions could not be satisfactorily answered and Stephen suffered what his father referred to as "the consequences of his actions." Stephen's father had asserted his position of power, and he would continue to do so for many years.

Day after day, Stephen was accused of crimes that he did not understand, but in time he accepted his guilt and hid his rage. Where, you might ask, were his mother and other family members? Stephen's mother was slow to respond to his needs and slow to provide him with even minimal protection. She did not physically abuse him, but she passively resisted meeting his most basic needs within any time frame but her own. Everyone in Stephen's family professed love for him, but none were willing to risk their own exclusion from the family by exposing this internal flaw to those outside of the family.

During his first year of life Stephen suffered both forced feeding and the withholding of food. He was jerked, pulled, dragged, thrown, and suspended upside down while being beaten about the head. When his father unexpectedly showed up in his room, Stephen cried out in terror, and his father would intermittently deprive him of oxygen until he stopped crying.

When Stephen was about 11 months old, his father decided to "make friends with him." For several weeks he took him on errands and on visits to family and friends. It was Stephen's job to sit with his father and to help present a picture of father/son love. This brief respite was not planned for Stephen's benefit, and it simply set him up for a deeper sense of betrayal. Like most children, he was not betrayed by strangers, but by close family members. This was allowed by the social forces within Stephen's community that adjudged that he was co-responsible for his father's acts, and this is what he, himself, believed.

Stephen grew up untreated and unhealed. He was artistically and academically gifted, but he did not finish high school. He turned to drugs and alcohol, and he drifted in and out of his family's life. He lied, stole, cheated, and betrayed the trust of all who trusted him. He had outbursts of rage that engendered fear in those who came to know him, and eventually he became an outcast both in his family and in society.

The patients I see often feel the depth of a pain that they cannot fully define. Children do experience pain, and if this pain is prolonged and/or goes untreated, it denies them access to the world. Their development of a self is stunted, and their desire somehow to heal their own lack of wholeness may drive them to the temporary wholeness that drugs and alcohol may appear to provide. Pain may also remain dormant for many years, or be manifested in numerous other ways, but it will not be forgotten.

Preventive healthcare is the communication of love and caring. It is a movement from a place of pain to an image of the possibility of a place in the world.

In the second half of her book Elaine Scarry introduces the concept of restoring and/or creating a world. She refers to this as the "making of the world," and pain and imagery, and the spectrum between these poles are explored. To restore one's place in the world there must be some sense of having a world to restore. When a child enters the world, he/she needs to be a partner in the creation of the world. If this does not occur, the child is likely to dwell in a place of pain and loneliness. When the necessary connections to explore one's own sense of being are lacking, early death or the creation of an inner world that serves to sever all connection with the outer world may occur. This produces a situation of tragedy, and the restoration and/or creation of a world may be impossible.

For a child to develop a world, he/she needs at least one person who joins him/her in the process of creating a world. There is a need to be both called out and to be introduced to the sensate world of images. Let us return for a moment to Elaine Scarry's writings on pain and imagination.

> It was noticed at an early point in this book that physical pain is exceptional in the whole fabric of psychic, somatic, and perceptual states for being the only one that has no object. Though the capacity to experience physical pain is as primal a fact about the human being as is the capacity to hear, to touch, to desire, to fear, to hunger, it differs from these events, and from every other bodily and psychic event, by not having an object in the external world. Hearing and touch are of objects outside the boundaries of the body, as desire is desire of x, fear is fear of y, hunger is hunger for z; but pain is not "of" or "for" anything—it is itself alone. . . .

The only state that is as anomalous as pain is the imagination. While pain is a state remarkable for being wholly without objects, the imagination is remarkable for being the only state that is wholly its objects. There is in imagining no activity, no "state," no experienceable condition or felt-occurrence separate from the objects: the only evidence that one is "imagining" is that imaginary objects appear in the mind. . . . pain and imagining are the "framing events" within whose boundaries all other perceptual, somatic, and emotional events occur; thus, between the two extremes can be mapped the whole terrain of the human psyche. . . . Imagining is, in effect, the ground of last resort. That is, should it happen that the world fails to provide an object, the imagination is there, almost on an emergency stand-by basis, as a last resource for the generation of objects. Missing, they will be made-up; and though they may sometimes be inferior to naturally occurring objects, they will always be superior to naturally occurring objectlessness.[5]

The images that we carry with us may serve to promote health or they may make it difficult to maintain our health. When I work with adults who are in pain, we work together to create healing images and to find healing images from the past that may promote healing.

Children are in the process of creating a world; so the most effective means of promoting health is to acknowledge their presence and concerns. In a recent *Los Angeles Times* article Lois Barclay Murphy, a child psychologist for many years, was acknowledged for the sensitivity and importance of her work.

What has earned her a place in the annals of psychological research is her fundamental belief in the importance of simply listening to children—following their lead rather than imposing adult standards on them.

Lois Barclay Murphy states:

Childbearing then is not just a matter of taking care of the baby and the young child—whether with a philosophy of permissiveness or of discipline—but of supporting the child's efforts to take care of himself.

As she reflects on a half century of work, what gives Murphy the most pride and satisfaction is the work that she did with the Head Start program for poor children in the 1960s.

Most vivid of all in her memory are those children—and their mothers—who changed, who were able to grow and achieve something they never would have achieved without Head Start. In particular, she remembers one mother, dirty and disheveled and without hope. "We put her on a committee on Head Start," Murphy said. Her appearance began to change. The woman went back to school, got her high-school equivalency certificate and began working. In other words," Murphy said, "she started feeling respected. She saw possibilities."[6]

In his article "Growing Up Mentally Fit," Lee Salk, Ph.D., provides excellent suggestions related to helping infants and young children develop the coping skills that are necessary if one is to dwell effectively in the spectrum between pain and imagination.

> How people deal with stresses during their adult years is determined to a great extent by what happens during infancy. . . . It is not only what happens during the early days, weeks and months of life, but oftentimes what does not happen during this early period that is important. . . . Infants subjected to long or frequent periods of stress do not become stronger and more effective in dealing with problems later on. Actually, they learn to use infantile methods for dealing with later stresses. . . . Infants and little babies who get cuddled a lot, whose parents try to meet all their needs during this period of great dependency, develop a sense of trust in others. Infants deprived of this kind of experience tend to lose trust in others and engage in very primitive behavior as a means of coping with stress—they tend to go off to sleep, tune out the world or engage in activities by themselves without any awareness of the outside world. . . . I think that it is crucially important for parents to show respect for the integrity of babies and children to help them to achieve a sense of self-esteem and the capacity to cope with frustration and stress. . . . It is important for the parents to show a sincere interest in the child's individuality in a way that helps the

child learn to function up to his or her potential in the demands of everyday life.[7]

What we learn from this and other articles is the fact that there is, in the prevention of chronic pain and chronic conditions, a beautiful simplicity that is attuned to the basic needs of each human life. When the needs of the infant and child are consistently ignored, the child is denied both confirmation and access to the world and may, in Maurice Friedman's words, settle for "the crumbs of life."

There is a third element that is important in Scarry's concept of "making and unmaking the world." Pain, at the one end of the spectrum, destroys the world and in the case of children may prevent the "making of the world." At the other end of the spectrum there is imagination which helps to make or restore the world. Pain and imagination represent the two extremes of a "self-contained loop," and it is the element of work that projects this loop into the world.

The placement of work within the spectrum will, however, determine whether it is closer to being pain or closer to being a creative task. Work that is meaningful and provides a sense of completion or satisfaction will be closer to the making and/or restoring of the world.

> That pain and the imagination are each other's missing intentional counterpart, and that they together provide a framing identity of man-as-creator within which all other intimate perceptual, psychological, emotional, and somatic events occur, is perhaps most succinctly suggested by the fact that there is one piece of language used—in many different languages—at once as a near synonym for pain, *and* as a near synonym for created object; and that is the word "work." The deep ambivalence of the meaning of "work" in Western civilization has often been commented upon, for it has tended to be perceived at once as pain's twin and as its opposite . . .
>
> Any sense that this duality is arbitrary dissolves when work is seen against the full array of intentional acts and objects; for work (like all the intentional states looked at above but to a much greater

degree than was apprehensible there) conforms to this same arrangement. The more it realizes and transforms itself in its object, the closer it is to the imagination, to art, to culture; the more it is unable to bring forth an object or, bringing it forth, is then cut off from its object, the more it approaches the condition of pain.

. . . Far more than any other intentional state, work approximates the framing events of pain and the imagination, for it consists of both an extremely embodied physical act (an act which, even in nonphysical labor, engages the whole psyche) and of an object that was not previously in the world, a fishing net or piece of lace where there had been none, or a mended net or repaired lace curtain where there had been only a torn approximation, or a sentence or a paragraph or a poem where there had been silence. Work and its "work" (or work and its object, its artifact) are the names that are given to the phenomena of pain and the imagination as they begin to move from being a self-contained loop within the body to becoming the equivalent loop now projected into the external world. It is through this movement out into the world that the extreme privacy of the occurrence (both pain and imagining are invisible to anyone outside the boundaries of the person's body) begins to be sharable [sic], that sentience becomes social and thus acquires its distinctly human form.[8]

I stated earlier in this chapter that the most basic element in the prevention of chronic pain is the need to love, nurture, and protect our children. If we look at work as a movement out into the world, it is important to recognize that each child must be given the tools to help him/her to accomplish the task of "making the world." This is not a solitary task. At every moment the child looks for confirmation and guidance.

If the child is continually punished and/or neglected, his/her ability to make a world is diminished or destroyed, and his/her work in the world becomes a source of pain. If, on the other hand, the child is provided with images of well being and reasonable tasks, he/she will feel a sense of accomplishment and empowerment. It is this early foundation that will, as mentioned earlier, affect each person's ability to cope with the physical and emotional injuries that occur throughout his or her lifetime.

The power of the healing partnership helps the child to create a world. The prevention of pain is based on recognizing the importance of each child's worth and his/her need to engage in making the world; dancing, singing, playing, drawing, speaking, grasping, releasing, throwing, putting together, taking apart, eating, crawling, touching, poking, and countless other activities help the child begin the process of moving out into the world. During this process there are many opportunities to help the child along his/her way, and to offer support to the parents. The elements of the healing partnership are present in both the prevention and treatment of chronic pain and chronic disorders.

Each child is a source of wonder, and when we see the beauty of a child who is nurtured and loved we also see the possibility of every child. In the case of Kai it is also possible to see the possibility of healing that arises from a healing partnership.

Kai

When Kai's parents decided to have their first child, they were surprised and pleased when the pregnancy occurred within a short period of time. They both shared the household tasks, and they looked forward to sharing the responsibility of caring for their child.

The pregnancy went well during the first four months, but then there were signs that Kai might arrive long before he was capable of living outside of the womb. Complete bed rest, sophisticated monitors, and medications were all recommended, and Kai's mother did what was necessary to protect his life. She also protected him by eating healthily, avoiding alcohol and caffeine, and by giving him light massages to communicate her love for him.

Kai was a family member long before his birthdate. Once it had been determined that he was a healthy male fetus his parents began the process of choosing a name for him. After a few weeks of exploration and debate he was named Kai, and from then on he was called by his name.

Kai was called into being before he was born. His parents showed us his sonogram pictures, and we felt as if his eyes met ours and saw beyond his own inner environment. Music, relaxation tapes, and his parents' voices were all a part of his inner world and added to his nurturing environment. Along with many others in his community, I hoped and prayed that he would be able to stay in this safe environment until he was capable of existing outside of the womb.

When Kai's weight was estimated to be at least 5½ pounds, he was considered a viable fetus. A week after this conclusion was reached the medication that had helped to keep him in the womb was decreased, and his mother was given exercises to help her prepare for the birth. Everything was in place, but the birth came sooner than was anticipated. There were unexpected complications and Kai was delivered by Caesarian section. He was a healthy five-pound, seven-ounce boy. The family and medical staff were both delighted and relieved by his healthy state.

Three hours after his birth Kai began to experience signs of respiratory distress. His mother was recovering from the effects of the surgery so his father was called in for a medical consultation. A new drug was available, but it had not been widely tested. This drug might prove Kai's only chance for recovery, but it was a high-risk situation. Distraught and with no other hope, Kai's father gave his permission to utilize the medication, but unfortunately there were adverse side effects. Kai was now in critical condition and had to be transferred to a more sophisticated treatment center. Kai's father accompanied him in the ambulance and stayed by his side for the next 16 hours. The prognosis was poor. If, by some miracle, Kai survived, he might suffer permanent disabilities that would severely affect his chances for a quality life. His father spoke to him, touched him, and agonized over wanting life for him, but not if it meant a greatly impaired life.

For 24 hours Kai's life hung in the balance, and then a miracle did occur. His condition stabilized and dramatically improved. A day later he was transferred back to the former hospital, and he was reunited with his mother. He remained in the hospital for 2 more weeks, and at least one of his parents was always with him. He learned to suck in nourishment from his bottle and began to gain weight. Kai was thriving and there were no signs that he would in any way suffer damaging effects from his ordeal.

Kai went home to a place of love and protection. His mother returned to part-time work, and his father stayed home and cared for him for the first 4 months. Later, both parents arranged work schedules that allowed some time for child-care responsibilities. Gradually they also increased other sources of child care.

Kai is a healthy, strong, alert, beautiful child. Each day he is called forth to be a part of life. He is introduced to colors, shapes, sounds, movements, and the many other elements of life. He is given support, reasonable limits and lots of love. He is creating a world, and he knows that he has a place in that world.

Someone once questioned whether Kai was suffering a panic attack when his respiratory distress began. "Could it be," they asked, "that the sudden separation from his mother and all that quieted and supported him was the source of his great distress?" I cannot answer this question, but I think that Kai's ability to heal was greatly enhanced by the healing partnership that existed within his family, and by the love that he was given before and after his birth.

One of the meanings of Kai's name is "singing heart." When I see Kai I find that he is indeed a loving, responsive infant, and he hums. Kai shows us the potential of every child, and every child deserves a singing heart.

Notes

1. Joan Borysenko, *Minding The Body, Mending the Mind* (Massachusetts: Addison-Wesley Publishing, 1987), cover statement.
2. Janny Scott, "Premature infants," *Los Angeles Times* (December 31, 1990).

3. Elaine Scarry, *The Body in Pain* (New York: Oxford University Press, 1985), p. 35.
4. Ibid., pp. 52–53.
5. Ibid., pp. 162, 165–166.
6. Sally Squires, "From mouths of babes, insights," *Los Angeles Times* (December 13, 1989), p. E20.
7. Lee Salk, "Growing up mentally fit," *Blue Print for Health—Blue Cross Association* (Illinois, 1974), pp. 18–25.
8. Elaine Scarry, *Body in Pain*, pp. 35.

CHAPTER 18

An Excellent Death

I took the title of this chapter from an article by Alice Walker. It is an article about excellence, the excellence of a healthy life and of a healthy death. A healthy life is sustained by the food that we eat, the environment that we live in, and the family and friends that support us and accept our support. Alice Walker states:

> America should have closed down and examined its every intention, institution, and law of the very first day that a black woman observed that the collard greens tasted like water. Or when the first person of any color observed that store bought tomatoes taste more like unripened avocados than like tomatoes.
>
> The flavor of food is one of the clearest messages the universe ever sends to human beings: and we have by now eaten poisoned warnings by the ton.[1]

The tasteless food that Alice Walker refers to is part of the cityscape that removes us from nature and the source of our food. Crowded together and yet lacking community, life itself may be as colorless as the food is tasteless. The greatest threat to our life energy may be the lack of a nurturing environment. Individual worth is diminished, and the core of one's being is atrophied. To have an excellent death, there must be an excellent life; not necessarily a life of material comfort, but certainly one of some personal comfort—the comfort of knowing that there is some loving constancy in life that calls out to your own individuality. This constancy is the thread that unites the possibility for excellence in life with the possibility of excellence in death. Alice Walker's article beautifully illustrates this point.

Some years ago as an adult I accompanied my mother to visit a very old neighbor who was dying a few doors down the street, and though she was no longer living in the country, the country style lingered. People like my mother were visiting her constantly, bringing food, picking up and returning laundry, or simply stopping by to inquire how she was feeling and to chat. Her house, her linen, her skin all glowed with cleanliness. She lay propped against pillows so that by merely turning her head she could watch the postman approach, friends and relatives arriving, and most of all, the small children playing beside the street, often in her yard, the sound of their play a lively music.

Sitting in the dimly lit, spotless room, listening to the lengthy but warm-with-shared-memories silences between my mother and Mrs. Davis was extraordinarily pleasant. Her white hair gleamed against her kissable black skin and her bed was covered with one of the most intricately patterned quilts I'd ever seen—a companion to the dozen or more she'd stored in a closet, which, when I expressed interest, she invited me to see.

I thought her dying one of the most reassuring events I'd ever witnessed. She was calm, she seemed ready, her affairs were in order. She was respected and loved. In short, Mrs. Davis was having an excellent death. A week later, when she had actually died, I felt this all the more because she had left, in me, the indelible knowledge that such a death is possible. And that cancer and nuclear annihilation are truly obscene alternatives. And surely, teaching this very vividly is one of the things an excellent death is supposed to do.

To die miserably of self-induced sickness is an aberration we take as normal; but it is crucial that we remember and teach our children that there are other ways.

For myself; for all of us, I want a death like Mrs. Davis's. When we will ripen and ripen further, richly as fruit, and then fall slowly into the caring arms of our friends and other people we know.

People who will remember the good days and the bad, the names of lovers and grandchildren, the time sorrow almost broke, the time friendship healed.

It must become a right of every person to die of old age. And if we secure this right for ourselves, we can, coincidentally, assure it for the planet. And that, as they say, will be excellence, which is, perhaps, only another name for health.[2]

This chapter is about the excellence that Alice Walker associates with health and "the right of every person to die of old age." This discussion takes us back to the work of Hans Selye and the adverse effects of chronic stress and/or chronic pain.

Chronic stress and/or chronic pain may not be direct causes of death, but they do cause wear and tear on the body, which leads to premature aging. They destroy the quality of life and may eventually destroy the will to live. The great medical advances of this century have increased the average life span of the majority of people in the United States. We do not so often die from germs and microbes, as from our own "voluntary, suicidal behavior." This behavior violates the natural laws that govern the aging process. The adaptation energy that sustains the quality of life is seriously depleted, and one exists without living.

In chemical terms one might view adaptation energy as the ability to remove the chemical scars of life. Each biological process leads to some chemical changes whose end-products are usually soluble or subject to destruction and elimination. Whenever this form of restoration is rapid, and recovery complete, our tissues undergo little change and we remain "young." However, an infinitesimally small percentage of all biologic reaction-products are insoluble, or at least less rapidly removable than their rate of deposition. The so-called "aging pigments," calcium deposits, cross-linked proteins, and many other products of biologic activity belong to this class. Mere excessive accumulation suffices to block the machinery. It could induce the changes we consider characteristic of aging by the mere presence of ever larger amounts of inert waste products and the consequent inability to produce indispensable vital ingredients at the proper rate.[3]

Much has been written about the causes and effects of stress, but the writings of Hans Selye provide us with the seminal work in this field. Selye points out that mainly we die because of the failure of one main part to function. We do not die as a whole, but rather because of the interdependency within the whole. To protect the whole of one's self, one must protect the individual parts. Selye presents the following quotient[4]:

$$\frac{\text{local stress in any one part}}{\text{total stress in the body}}$$

In order to break the cycle of stress and/or pain there must be diversion. Diversion helps to divert both the mental and physical stress that accumulates over time, but by removing our awareness of pain it may add stress to stress. When we fail to heed the warning signs that signal an overload on one or more body systems, the sources of our life energy will be taxed. If, however, we do not sufficiently tax the sources of our adaptation energy, we may never begin to know the limits of our own individual being. "It is only in the heat of stress that individuality can be perfectly molded."[5] What is important here is to realize that adaptation energy is ours to spend, and that it is, from the beginning of life, influenced by our heredity, the events of our life, and our personal choices.

We do not have control over our heredity or many of the events of our life, but we do have the opportunity to make our own personal choices. This brings me back to my professional beginnings and explains, in part, my interest in the field of chronic stress and chronic pain.

For over fifteen years I worked with teachers, parents, and children in one of the largest school districts in the country. I was, during those years, a classroom teacher, health coordinator, articulation coordinator, and student counselor. When you work in a school you see, on a daily basis, the adverse effects of chronic stress and chronic pain. Parents, teachers, administrators, and students are all under stress, but it is the student population that is most in need of support and guidance, and it is the children and young adults who suffer the greatest loss when the adult population is unable to meet their needs. Children need to know that they have the capacity to enhance their health and that their own personal choices can make a difference. Without guidance and support it is difficult to discover one's own capacity for managing stress and pain. It is not unusual to discount children's symptoms of chronic stress, chronic pain, and/or chronic illnesses, and sometimes children with these symptoms are labeled as malingerers or as having behavioral problems. Busy parents may resent being bothered by their children's chronic complaints, and schools may insist that a child stay in class unless he/she has a temperature or some other obvious sign of illness.

Children are not immune to the health problems that plague our adult population. They too suffer from headaches, ulcers, depression, allergies, fatigue, sleep disturbance, anxiety, cancer, loneliness, and most other stress-related maladies that affect the adult population. Children may arrive at school hungry, tired, cold, ill, angry, sad, frightened, anxious, and/or suffering from any number of other conditions that make it difficult for them to concentrate and to accomplish what is asked of them. They may live in a very stressful home situation, and their neighborhood may be a source of additional stress. Many children receive only minimal parenting and suffer from economic deprivation, and the school may provide their only source of constancy and support. Teachers, however, cannot meet the needs of every child in their classroom. It is an impossible task given the number of students that most teachers must work with each day. Each child and young adult needs to be called out as a person and to gain a sense of their own worth. A society that does not foster the elements of the healing partnership sets the stage for increased stress, illness, and pain. Healing occurs in partnership and, as Martin Buber states, "Only as a partner can a person be perceived as an existing wholeness." When the "mob" mentality becomes the norm, the individual's voice is lost and with it the partnership of existence.

The Joy and the Pride of Teaching a Class, Not a Mob

I am sitting at my desk at Bell High School, reading compositions written by my 9th-grade English class. My students have written essays in the form of news reports. Their topic: the death of Romeo Montague and Juliet Capulet. I am bursting with pride and anger.

No "gifted" students these. They are labeled "average." Their essays are among the best I've ever seen for that grade level and I've been looking for 15 years.

How is it possible to get such superior work out of "average" kids?

The answer is that there are only 13 kids in the class. (How did I get such a small class? A scheduling fluke.) A class of 35 to 40 "average" 9th-graders would never produce such high-quality work. With such big numbers the teacher has to spend as much time dealing with behavioral problems as he or she does teaching. There is virtually no time for individualized instruction, and the increased time spent on paper-grading means proportionally less time for creative lesson preparation.

This is nothing new. Everyone connected with education knows the effect of class size on student accomplishment. And that's why I'm angry. Piled on my desk is the clearest evidence I've ever seen of what my colleagues and I can accomplish, given a reasonable chance to reach students' minds. Why are we not given a chance? How many uninspired imaginations and undereducated intellects are we going to shove out the schoolhouse door, clutching worthless academic diplomas in their hands, for a march into substandard jobs, adding to the list of the economically deprived.

A few days ago I was stopped on the school quad and informed that because of the small number of students this class will be closed next month. I need to rush and teach them all I can before they become lost in the mobs that populate our other classrooms. How will anyone reach them?

Of Juan Aguilar I speak, and Armando Gutierrez, and Graciela Gonzales; Ron Washington, Shawna Jackson and Han Nguyen, victims of overcrowded classrooms and assembly-line education, an oxymoron in any teacher's terms.

Wake up, America. Their future is our future.

—Joel Littauer

Joel Littauer is a mentor–teacher for the Los Angeles public schools and author of "Manual of Motivational Strategies"
(JAG Publications, 1989).[6]

Video games, television, movies, and overcrowded classrooms cannot provide the personal response that every child needs to develop a sense of personal worth. Each person that touches a child's life may help to ease his or her transition from one stage of life to another. The teachers, teaching aides, bus drivers, volunteers, office personnel, administrators, crossing guards, school nurses, and all others who participate in the child's world have the opportunity to recognize the uniqueness of each child and to help that child to develop his/her own voice.

We live in a society that is not kind and gentle to its children. There is a great need to foster a caring community that recognizes the needs of children and young adults. The effects of chronic stress, chronic pain, and chronic illness rob one of an excellent life and an excellent death.

Sweden may be the only country in the world with a systematic, basic mental- and relaxation-training program in their school system. This system is based on six years of research and has served as a model program throughout the world. The program is called *"Relaxation Training for Youth"*[7] and there are two major areas of training. The first area of training is called *"Basic Relaxation Training for Youth,"* and the second area of training is called *"Development of Basic Capacities."* The training program includes a teacher's manual and two tapes that guide the children through the program. I have selected certain passages from the teacher's manual to provide a sense of both the theory and the practical application of the program.

Introduction

Relaxation can be seen as nature's own medicine. It builds on inherent abilities which can maintain this capacity and develop it. . . . Relaxation is not only the least complicated medicine to inhibit or remove stress, but it is also the most effective and natural method of all. As small children all of us could completely relax and become as limp as a rag doll. How many of us can now do this?

Now, in Sweden, the school authorities are helping growing youngsters to maintain and develop their own inherent abilities to relax and "heal" themselves . . . But Swedes are not content to rest with relaxation but instead regard relaxation as only the first step towards helping individuals more fully develop their innate but often latent abilities. Already a project has been carried out introducing concentration training into schools and a more thorough, systematic training program is being suggested. This new program is to help growing children, the future adults and maintainers of the world, to maintain and develop their own positive capacities which all people have as children but most of us lose by adulthood.

Theory of Relaxation

We try to contend with our uneasiness, our tension and stress with their accompanying neurotic and psychosomatic conditions. Often we are attracted to use more or less complicated (and frequently expensive) methods, while we easily forget the easiest, most natural methods. Relaxation seems to be nature's own tranquilizer. "The most difficult thing about relaxation methods," the Australian psychiatrist Ainslie Meares says, "is that they are so simple." The solutions to most of our problems are already inside of us and all we have to do is to find a method to release these self-healing powers, giving them an opportunity to heal and restore our normal balance.

General Effects of Relaxation—Effects on Behavior

When you begin to practice relaxation, you usually sit or lie still and perhaps close your eyes. For a person on the outside, this can appear to be a passive and sleeplike state. However this is not a necessary characteristic for relaxation and dissociation. After a period of training most people can attain a decrease in muscle tone, a mental effect of calm and certainty and a dissociation from disturbing factors even while they are directly engaged in an activity. Training is directed at teaching an ability which you can always have with you and quickly use in everyday life without needing to withdraw from the situation in which you find yourself. In other words, there is no need to change your outer behavior in order to relax and reduce tension.

General Uses—Images

One of the main principles upon which self-control through mental imagery is based is the following assumption: Our nervous system has difficulty in distinguishing between a situation we imagine vividly and a real situation. We can eliminate the difference between imaginary situations and reality by making the images as real as possible. In this way we can gain new experiences for ourselves and store them in our memories . . . In a relaxed state our imagination and picture-creation ability (right brain) are improved and our images become more and more real. Imagery training should therefore be combined with relaxation.

Specific Areas of Use

All people these days have experienced some uneasiness and tension. This feeling is often diffuse and therefore difficult to describe. It can be intense or weak. Sometimes it is felt only as a sort of unrest or nervousness at work or with friends. You notice perhaps that you are more easily irritated, impatient and touchy. You may have difficulty in concentrating or perhaps a creeping feeling that something is wrong, but you do not know just what it is. Anxiety and tension appear in how you speak or sleep (or do not sleep). Some people have other problems that they do not realize arise from anxiety . . .

Some people are so accustomed to tension and anxiety that they cannot even imagine that things could be otherwise. Others who suffer from these problems try to find a solution on their own. The most common types of attempted solutions consist of some form of "determination" ("take hold of yourself," "pull yourself together," "just try harder"). These are very poor methods which often lead to increased tension instead of less. It has been shown that the more and the harder you try to get rid of anxiety the more it increases . . . Relaxation techniques are a method which, on the one hand, can give a direct easing of the symptoms and, on the other hand, can be combined with other more long-range treatments . . . It has been shown that deep relaxation induces a mental relaxation which includes a feeling of calmness and certainty. Scientific research has shown that deep relaxation combats stress and anxiety. Or, in other words, it is very difficult to feel unrest and fear or have negative feelings when the muscles in your body are completely relaxed.

Care and Maintenance of Childlike Capacities

Children have several valuable primitive qualities which grow or decline in their transition to adulthood. Children, for example, have a good imagination and powers of intense involvement and concentration, as well as senses of curiosity and creativity coupled with an ability to laugh at many different types of things . . .

The first part of this booklet describes the project of relaxation training in Swedish schools from 1976 to 1984. It includes instructions for children, teachers and parents as well as a summary of research results. Part 2 takes up the first attempts to introduce confidence training in one school. It also introduces a program which includes six other childlike capacities—the 7 C's for short.

C-1 Confidence

The emphasis on a good self-image as a base for good goal-images and good performance in school, sport and other activities makes it especially important to obtain early confidence training . . . For most people confidence is a result of what has happened to them or more precisely their interpretation of events. A bad start in any area often leads to one or more vicious circles that can continue throughout the individual's entire life. Confidence training aims at turning this around. By developing a good self-image early, independent external events, increased self-confidence helps steer and direct future events and one's interpretation of them. "Circles" will start but they will be "positive" instead of "vicious."

C-2 Commitment

Motivation is the core of life. It is the answer to why we do or do not do things. If we were boats on the sea of life then we could say that motivation is the wind that fills our sails as well as our rudder. It gives us the thrust to get going as well as deciding our direction.

Goal setting: In order for goals to be stimulating and engaging they ought to be self-selected. They may be suggested by parents, teachers or other key persons but it is important for kids—as for adults—not only to accept but also to feel for goals—to accept them as their own. Goals should be concrete, specific and controlled by the individual. Based on this principal, competition ought to be defined not as a struggle between individuals but as a struggle within a person to reach goals which he or she controls.

Goal-integration: If motivation training is limited to analytical procedures, then there is a great risk that motivation training and goal-setting will become but another stress factor in life. Therefore, in order to make goals into a stimulating and energy force, goals must be programmed or integrated into one's person. Such integration is best done in a deeply relaxed state.

C-3 Calmness

Feelings of calmness usually accompany muscular relaxation. In this third program, however, the feeling of calmness is intensified by the use of exhaling as a trigger . . . The purpose is to give the person a tool which can be used in any situation where he or she wants to relax or calm down, as for example, before giving a short speech in class. The individual learns to calm down quickly by taking a few deep breaths.

C-4 Creativity

Creativity is another capacity which is easiest to use and develop when relaxed. This program builds on children's natural sense of curiosity and imagination. It is meant to help the individual have courage to maintain and develop their innate abilities in these areas. This again is done while in a deeply relaxed state during which the pupil uses his/her imagination.

C-5 Cheerfulness

This program, as in the earlier programs, is built upon children's innate abilities. Small children can laugh and be happy for the smallest of things in the right circumstances. They can laugh at almost anything, including what they do themselves. Very quickly, however, we learn to see "seriously" most of what we do and lose much of our sense of humor, especially the ability to laugh at ourselves and be spontaneously happy.

C-6 Concentration

Concentration involves both learning to be more attentive to a limited area (focusing) and learning to ignore or pay less attention to other irrelevant stimuli (dissociation). This or rather these abilities are developed during this sixth program.

C-7 Control

Mostly we are taught to take control by gritting our teeth and trying harder or in other words by tensing up. This seventh program teaches how to take control in a more positive relaxed manner instead of tensing up.

We are controlled to a great extent by events around us that have entered our subconscious and over which we no longer have control. Therefore, we at times may become aggressive and angry or perhaps blush when we don't want to, for example. This program helps the individual to gain more control in such situations.

The results of Sweden's relaxation-training program for youth demonstrates the benefits of a program that focuses on helping young people enhance their own innate capacity for handling stress. Much of a child's education is focused on diminishing their capacity for deep relaxation, and there is little emphasis on the development of their "basic childlike capacities." Children are taught to "tune out" their body signals. They learn to sit for increasingly long periods of time, to eat, drink, and eliminate according to bell schedules, and to suppress both their joy and their sorrow. The larger the classes, the less room for individuality, and the personal response is silenced in favor of conformity.

My work with adult patients has given me the opportunity to appreciate more fully the importance of deep relaxation and the enhancement of "childlike capacities." When I work with a patient, I am addressing his or her symptoms in relation to family, friends, and workplace. Our task is to work together to reawaken the patient's own capacity for healing and to develop an appreciation of his or her "basic childlike capacities."

The child is taught by the adult world both directly and indirectly how to conduct his/her life. We cannot give each child the constancy that Alice Walker writes about in her article, but we can help each child to develop the resources to deal with a changing society. Excellent health comes from being able to relax and from nurturing our "basic childlike capacities." It is the adult's task to help each child reach adulthood with these capacities intact. When this occurs, there is a greater opportunity for excellent health and an excellent death.

Notes

1. Alice Walker, "On excellence," *Ms. Magazine* (January, 1985), p. 53.
2. Ibid., pp. 53–56.
3. Hans Selye, *The Stress of Life* (New York: McGraw-Hill, 1976), p. 431.
4. Ibid., p. 416.
5. Ibid., p. 433.
6. Joel Littauer, "The joy and pride of teaching a class," *Los Angeles Times* (Editorial, January, 1991).
7. Sven Setterlind, Lars-Eric Uneståhl, and Bob Kaill, *Relaxation Training for Youth* (Sweden: Stress Management Center, 1986), pp. 5–21.

CHAPTER 19

A Biofeedback Treatment Protocol

Within the last 10 years it has become increasingly evident that the possibilities for self-regulation are only beginning to be realized and that many questions remain unanswered. The fields of psychophysiology and psychoneuroimmunology have expanded the concept of self-regulation and provided us with a glimpse of the human potential for healing.

We have moved from viewing the patient as a passive recipient of health care to the opposite extreme, so far, in fact, that we fear that the patient may begin to feel fully responsible for his or her own illness and recovery. What is important in the healing partnership is the sharing of responsibility and the realization that healing is facilitated within the healing partnership.

In this chapter I have attempted to present a treatment protocol with an emphasis on the utilization of the two biofeedback modalities that are commonly used to help patients decrease the symptoms of chronic pain or a chronic condition. I have placed this chapter toward the end of the book because there is a danger of seeing the treatment protocol as something that can be routinely carried out by a trained technician. I find that the visual and audio biofeedback signals help patients to understand better the concept of self-regulation and to gain a sense of their own capacity to decrease their symptoms. Eventually most patients learn that they can obtain satisfactory results without the use of biofeedback equipment, but we all utilize certain forms of biofeedback to assess our own state of well-being.

I generally utilize one or more biofeedback modalities when I treat a patient, and I may monitor the muscle-tension levels in at least three or four different sites. I use very basic biofeedback equipment, and at all times it is the patient, not an established treatment plan, that dictates the treatment protocol. There are those who believe that the level of technology makes a basic difference, but I believe that the relationship between the therapist and the patient is the most important factor in the healing process.

There are numerous biofeedback intake questionnaires. I have provided examples of those that I have found helpful in my own practice (see pp. 269–271). I also have access to each patient's medical chart and to psychological evaluations, but I generally focus on the patient's own voice.

Joyce

Joyce was self-referred for headaches. She had a mixed head-ache pattern of both muscle-contraction and vascular (migraine) headaches. She had been medically treated without satisfactory results and stated that she had decided "to give biofeedback a try." When asked about her symptoms, she stated:

> I seldom have a day without a headache, but the symptoms vary in intensity. The migraines are the worst, and they generally occur about every four or five weeks, and really knock me out. The other headaches occur almost everyday, but there isn't an exact pattern. They do tend to occur more often in the late afternoon, but sometimes I wake up with a headache or get one in the evening. I seldom miss work because of a headache, but I am tired of having headaches and tired of trying to control them with medications.

During this first session I learned that Joyce's migraine head-

BIOFEEDBACK INTAKE QUESTIONNAIRE

NAME				DATE	
MEDICAL RECORD NUMBER				DIAGNOSIS	
ADDRESS					
HOME PHONE NUMBER			HOME PHONE NUMBER		
AGE	SEX	OCCUPATION			
MARITAL STATU		REFERRING DOCTOR			

NAME OF PRESCRIPTION MEDICATION	DATE STARTED	DOSAGE

NAME OF NONPRESCRIPTION MEDICATION	DATE STARTED	DOSAGE

CHECK THOSE WORDS WHICH BEST DESCRIBE YOU:

☐ calm   ☐ satisfied   ☐ restless   ☐ perfectionistic

☐ energetic ☐ lonely   ☐ nervous   ☐ driving

☐ easygoing ☐ depressed   ☐ anxious   ☐ fatigued

☐ frustrated ☐ tense   ☐ critical   ☐ worrisome

	YES	NO	SPECIFY TYPE AND AMOUNT
CAFFEINE CONSUMPTION (coffee, tea, colas)			
SMOKING HABITS			
ALCOHOL CONSUMPTION			
PHYSICAL EXERCISE			

CHECK THE SITUATIONS WHICH ARE CURRENTLY STRESSFUL:

☐ Parents   ☐ Work   ☐ Symptoms

☐ Children   ☐ School   ☐ Sex

☐ Spouse   ☐ Social Life   ☐ Finances

☐ Other relatives ☐ Other: _____

BIOFEEDBACK INTAKE QUESTIONNAIRE

NAME: _____ DATE: _____

MEDICAL RECORD NUMBER: _____ DIAGNOSIS: _____

ADDRESS: _____

HOME PHONE: _____ BUSINESS PHONE: _____

AGE: _____ SEX: _____ OCCUPATION: _____

MARITAL STATUS: _____ REFERRING DOCTOR: _____

APPROXIMATE DATE OF ONSET OF PAIN: _____

SYMPTOM: _____

FREQUENCY:

☐Seldom   ☐Monthly   ☐Weekly   ☐Several times per week   ☐Daily   ☐Several times per day

INTENSITY:

☐Mild   ☐Discomforting   ☐Distressing   ☐Horrible   ☐Excruciating

DURATION:

☐Seconds or minutes   ☐Hours   ☐Days   ☐Constant waxes and wanes   ☐Constant unchanging

Put a dot in the center of your pain. Shade in lightly the *areas* affected by pain.

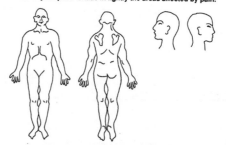

WHAT KINDS OF THINGS RELIEVE OR REDUCE YOUR PAIN? _____

_____

WHAT KINDS OF THINGS INCREASE YOUR PAIN? _____

_____

BIOFEEDBACK INTAKE QUESTIONNAIRE

NAME: _____ DATE: _____

Put a dot in the center of your pain. Shade in lightly the areas affected by pain.

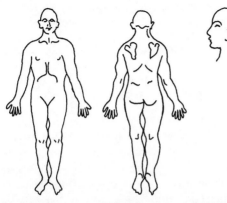

CHECK THOSE SYMPTOMS WHICH YOU EXPERIENCE FREQUENTLY:

____Throbbing headaches	____Itching	____Burping
____Dull, aching headaches	____Excessive need to urinate	____Gasiness
____Soreness of muscles	____Stuttering	____Acid stomach
____Tightness in jaw	____Voice quavering or shaking	____Difficulty falling asleep
____Grinding or clenching teeth	____Shakiness	____Difficulty staying asleep
____Weakness in parts of body	____Tightness in throat	____Bad dreams
____Twitches, tics, and spasms	____Constipation	____Worrying or ruminating thoughts
____Faintness or dizziness	____Diarrhea	____Difficulty concentrating
____Fatigue	____Abdominal pain or distress	____Your mind goes blank
____Lower back pains	____Tightness in stomach	____Difficulty remembering things
____Pains in heart or chest	____Nausea or vomiting	____Loss of interest in things
____Rapid heartbeat	____Poor appetite	____Easily annoyed or irritated
____Trouble getting your breath	____Overeating	____Uncontrollable outbursts
____Feeling tense or nervous	____Difficulty in swallowing	____Easily crying
____Cold extremities	____Heartburn	____Extreme fear of places or events
____Sweaty palms	____Regurgitation of food or fluid	____Feeling fearful

aches had started during her late teens but were not directly connected to her menses. She was now 32 years old, unmarried, lived alone, was not close to her family, and liked her work as a computer programmer. She earned an excellent income, enjoyed time with her friends, and liked the company of her dog and two cats. When asked how long she had been suffering from the muscle contraction headaches, she stated:

> Up until ten years ago I would sometimes have an occasional tension (muscle-contraction) headache, but I could take something like aspirin and decrease the symptoms within an hour. The headaches crept up on me over the past ten years, and I kept trying to ignore them, but now it is impossible. The funny thing is that the migraine headaches have remained about the same in frequency and intensity, and now I am more concerned about the tension headaches than the migraines—except, of course, when I have a migraine headache.

During our initial conversation I learned that Joyce often worked overtime, and did not exercise on a regular basis, but did like to camp and hike during her vacations. She was pleasant and did not appear to be in any distress during this first meeting. When asked about her condition, she stated that she had a very slight headache but did not have any other symptoms. She described herself as calm, energetic, perfectionistic, and sometimes driven. Joyce did not drink colas, she had one or two cups of coffee a day, did not smoke, and seldom drank alcohol. She was currently stressed by her parents (if they contacted her), her work (she tended to work long hours), her symptoms, and her finances (she was earning more money than she had ever expected to earn, and her affluence was a source of stress).

For several sessions I utilized the electromyograph (EMG) to help Joyce to reduce her upper-body tension levels. When the muscles exhibit elevated levels of tension during rest, it indicates a source of chronic tension. I monitored her upper-back muscles, neck and shoulder areas, forehead (frontalis), and the muscles of her jaw. We discussed ways to decrease eye tension and to utilize breathing techniques to reduce upper-body tension levels. On a scale of one to ten Joyce's highest levels of tension were over the frontalis and registered between 3.0 and 3.5. When she learned to reduce her jaw tension and to relax her eye tension, she brought this level down to a low of 1.5. I explained to her that it would not be normal to maintain a relaxed state throughout the day, but that the same is true of maintaining high levels of tension throughout the day. Ordinarily, a level of tension between 2.0 and 2.5 is considered a moderately low level of tension, and a tension level below 2.0 is considered a low level of tension. But this is not a standard that is accepted by all biofeedback therapists.

The EMG measures the electrical current that is produced by the muscle that is being monitored. During a time of rest the output should be low. But when a muscle or muscle group becomes chronically tense, the output is high, and the work load is inappropriate for the amount of work being done. This is a waste of one's resources, and it also contributes to chronic stress and chronic pain. The rhythm of the body is one of tense–relax, and when this rhythm is broken it exerts a stress that is communicated within the body as a whole.

Sometimes a patient will experience a dramatic reduction in his or her symptoms after only one or two sessions of biofeedback therapy. For a lasting effect the patient needs to incorporate what is being learned during the session into everyday life, and to generalize his or her ability to decrease the tension levels over one particular muscle group. EMG electrodes monitor surface muscle tension, and the ability to elicit a generalized relaxation response is important.

Joyce did not experience an immediate decrease in her symptoms, but she was becoming more aware of her habitual patterns of holding tension in the neck, shoulders, and facial area. When a pattern of tension becomes habitualized, it is not recognized and/or associated with the pain or discomfort that eventually surfaces. Then, too, some pain is referred pain, and it may be difficult to recognize the relationship between the pain itself and the actual source of the pain. This is especially true of back injuries, but temporomandibular joint (TMJ) disorders may also cause pain and/or discomfort that will appear to be unrelated to the primary source of the problem. Headaches, dizziness, ringing in the ears, facial pain, and other problems are often related to this common disorder.

I asked Joyce to practice "mini-exercises" off and on throughout the day so that she would begin to reduce her upper-body tension levels. These mini exercises included using her breathing to reduce facial tension, short tense–relax exercises for the neck and shoulders, consciously relaxing the eyes and masseter muscles from time to time, and moving and stretching whenever she had the chance to do so. I encouraged her to take time for lunch and a short walk everyday. Joyce worked a 50- to 60-hour work week. It is difficult to reduce symptoms if a connection with nature and diversity is lacking. We discussed the fact that she had other options and that it would be possible for her to plan short weekend trips. This would provide an opportunity for hiking and a total break from her work.

Joyce was beginning to have a decrease in her muscle-contraction headaches, and she had not yet had a vascular headache. I continued to monitor her upper-body tension levels, but I also introduced the blood-flow (temperature) feedback. This is a standard treatment modality for migraine headaches, but it is also a primary tool for general relaxation and to combat various other disorders. Except for the hands and feet, internal and external body temperatures remain about the same unless there is a traumatic injury or illness. The core temperature is usually about 99° F, and the external body temperature is slightly cooler. I have seen many patients who are chronically stressed, and their hand temperature is often in the low eighties. This is especially true of female patients. Migraine headaches are vascular headaches, and a drop in hand temperature is a warning sign that indicates the vascular tension that usually precipitates a migraine headache is occurring. I do not emphasize learning to warm the hands to abort a headache, but rather to utilize warming techniques to prevent migraine headaches.

It was not easy for Joyce to warm her hands so I covered her with a light blanket. She had become accustomed to her cool hands, and I wanted her to experience what it felt like to have warm extremities. Her pre-session finger temperature readings were in the low eighties and her post-session readings were in the low nineties. We worked on exercises that emphasized feelings of being heavy and warm, and I also introduced relaxing images. It takes time to relax the smooth muscles of the vascular system, but this is an excellent way to attain a deep state of relaxation.

Within 5 weeks Joyce's pre-session EMG levels were decreased, and she was able to maintain a low tension level throughout the session. She reported that she was having decreased tension headache symptoms but that she had suffered a migraine headache that had occurred over the weekend. It is not unusual for a vascular headache to occur after a week of hard work. Some patients feel punished for relaxing but it is often part of the "let down" phenomenon of the migraine headache pattern. With Joyce, as well as other patients, there is a need to explore one's own patterns. Diet, specific triggers, muscle tension, vascular tension, head injuries, extreme stress, and numerous other factors may contribute to an individual's headache pattern.

During the next month I continued to emphasize upper-body relaxation, temperature training, and the development of imagery skills. I gave Joyce some home practice tapes and some finger sensors that indicated changes in her hand temperature. This was still another way to help her to tune into the subtle body changes that contributed to her headache symptoms. Eventually, Joyce developed her own personal relaxation image. She was able to close her eyes, take a deep breath, exhale her chronic tension, and imagine her own personal relaxation image while she maintained relaxed breathing. This was a short exercise that provided a moment of deep relaxation. Joyce was beginning to understand her symptoms, and she was pleased by her progress. She was having fewer muscle-contraction headaches, and the intensity and duration of her migraine headaches had decreased. She had gone 6 weeks without having had a vascular headache, and she was now much more aware of the contributing factors. Joyce decided when it was time for her to continue working by herself, but we did schedule two follow-up sessions. She knew that she was not "cured," but she was aware of her own resources and her capacity for self-regulation. Joyce called me about a year after her final biofeedback session. She had purchased a house in a semi-rural area and she was able to do most of her work in her home computer center. She was taking daily walks, pacing herself, and enjoying her "almost headache-free existence."

During the last 10 years I have utilized specific biofeedback instrumentation for sphincter control, bladder control, and blood-pressure monitoring. To a lesser degree I have monitored sweat gland activity with the GSR (galvanic skin response) and brain-wave activity with the EEG (electroencephalograph). I have also met with patients who were uncomfortable with use of biofeedback equipment, and we have explored other ways for them to develop self-regulation skills. What is most important is the patient/therapist relationship, for that is what is most beneficial for the patient.

There is a great deal of controversy about the benefits of biofeedback therapy and this is especially true when there is clinical evidence that a patient has benefited from biofeedback therapy. The following article vividly illustrates this point:

> Never mind the electrodes taped to the little girl's shoulders. Or the two red sensors stuck to her left index finger and palm. Or the band of black elastic around her waist.
>
> Instead, in a basement room at Children's Hospital of Orange County, 6 year old Cory Barger stared at a video monitor that showed her muscle tension, perspiration, and breathing as bright, geometric designs.
>
> "Keep your shoulders quiet, Cory. Relax," technician Barbara Farber advised. And Cory let her shoulders fall. She took a breath. On the screen, blocks of pink, yellow and green turned to dazzling blue. "Wow," Cory says softly.
>
> The solemn-faced girl in the red Minnie Mouse dress was

practicing a relaxation technique called biofeedback that she uses often to control pain.

In remission from leukemia, Cory must have spinal taps every six weeks. But until she learned biofeedback, the needle jabs were agonizing. Each time, five nurses—or sometimes, four nurses and Cory's mother—had to hold down the often screaming 40-pound girl.

But since she began biofeedback last November, Cory has walked calmly to the spinal punctures, positioned herself on the table, and held her body still, concentrating on relaxing. "It makes my pokes not hurt too much," she explained.

Introduced in the late 1960s and still controversial, biofeedback is mental training that lets people gain control over involuntary bodily functions.

By wearing electronic sensors that "feed back" data on temperature, respiration or muscle tension to a biofeedback video monitor, patients discover ways of relaxing.

When an electrode is wrapped around a finger, for instance, the video screen will display the patient's temperature, sometimes as a wavering line. But by experimenting with ways of easing tension—breathing deeply, for instance, or imagining a quiet walk on the beach—a patient can gradually learn to make the temperature line rise. And slowly he has learned a simple method of relaxing—that of warming his hands.

Again, when an electrode is placed on a patient's shoulders, bright colors on the biofeedback monitor may indicate that the patient's shoulder muscles are tense. But by studying the monitor and trying to change the colors on the screen to ones that indicate relaxation, a patient can learn how to ease the tension.

Though the high-tech procedure was designed for adults, across the nation many psychologists and pediatricians now use biofeedback with children, a few as young as 2.

Not only does it help youngsters like Cory who need frequent, painful medical procedures but also, doctors at Children's Hospital and many other pediatric hospitals say, it can help treat a long list of disorders—from anxiety, migraine headaches and fiercely itching eczema to arthritis, attention deficit disorder, and a neurological syndrome called Raynaud's Disease.

In addition, Children's Hospital psychologist Frank Carden said, his staff uses biofeedback to "retrain" children with asthma and cystic fibrosis—improving their lung function by showing them how to breathe using the diaphragm, not the chest. A recent Children's Hospital study of 26 cystic fibrosis patients, ages 10 to 41, showed that those whose breathing was "retrained" with biofeedback improved lung function by 38% to 100% and would probably show long-term benefits, including fewer respiratory infections.

The list of uses for biofeedback goes on.

At the Hargitt Elementary School in Norwalk, counselor Micki East, uses biofeedback sensors and a computer game called "Stack Attack" to show first-through-seventh graders how their bodies react to stress.

In Tulsa, Okla., psychologist William Finley has created a patented biofeedback device to stop bed-wetting. And in Florida, at the University of Miami Medical Center, doctors use biofeedback to teach brain-damaged children and adults to move paralyzed limbs. With sensors attached to immobile arms or legs, patients try to move while the monitor shows if the muscle has received a signal from the brain.

Explained Dr. Bernard Brucker, a co-director of the Miami Project to Cure Paralysis: "We're teaching people to be more efficient at using the cells of the brain."

For all the enthusiasm, some doctors remain deeply skeptical about biofeedback, some suggesting that it is a modern form of snake oil. Many more are cautious, suggesting it may work for a few psychosomatic ailments but that most of the time, simple relaxation techniques may work just as well.

"It's of unproven scientific validity overall," said Ira Lott, chairman of pediatrics at UC Irvine School of Medicine. "In rare instances, biofeedback may help, but I would not recommend it as a prophylactic treatment in general."

Children's Hospital in Los Angeles rarely uses it, said its head of behavioral sciences, psychologist Michael Dolgin.

"A lot of people feel you can get just as good results with other techniques like hypnosis," he said. Still, some of Dolgin's private patients, especially youngsters with headaches, learn biofeedback. The technique teaches children to dilate blood vessels and ease their pain, said Dolgin, who believes it can give them a sense of mastery over their bodies.

One of the most negative reports on biofeedback came in 1987 when a committee of the National Research Council in Washington said there was no proof that it could relieve stress.

That finding still appears correct, said several committee members, including USC psychology professor Gerald Davison. He acknowledged that biofeedback research with paralyzed patients appears promising but said he still doubted many other claims made for the technique, which he described as "impressive gimmickry."

Biofeedback advocates counter angrily that the NRC study was uninformed, misleading and misstated the research.

Overall, the medical establishment has been quick to find fault with the technique, noted a biofeedback pioneer Judith Green.

"The sad story is we [biofeedback practitioners] don't get a lot of referrals" from doctors, said the Greely, Colorado, psychologist. "When a child shows up at the pediatrician's with a migraine, they think drugs. Or hyperactivity? They think Ritalin . . . But I think doctors are becoming more educated, more interested in mind–body therapies."

Cory's mother Barbara Burns said she might not have believed the claims about biofeedback either—if she hadn't seen it help her daughter.

After Cory was diagnosed with leukemia in April, 1987—immediately enduring three or four bone marrow aspirations that first week—Burns said she started searching desperately for some sort of pain management for her little girl.

"Our vet manages pain" with Cory's pony, Burns said. Before he gives the pony a shot, he loops a 10-inch chain around the animal's lip, twists it tightly "and the pony falls asleep."

"I thought, my God, if you can do that for horses they ought to be able to find a place on a human being" that would still the pain, Burns said. "But [the doctors] didn't have any suggestions."

So, for two years the situation didn't change. About every 12 weeks, Cory would have a spinal and each time, she would scream and have to be held down.

For a while, "they used to sedate her . . . a very painful poke in the leg and sometimes a poke in the hip to numb the area," Burns said. "But those would hurt so much." And sometimes the sedation, a form of "twilight sleep," would make Cory "wild."

Burns said she decided to join nurses in holding her flailing, screaming daughter during the five-minute-long puncture when she discovered, after one procedure, that Cory bore fingernail scratches from being pinned down. At 4½, Cory "made the decision that she didn't want to take the sedatives anymore," said Burns. "So the doctors suggested, 'Let's try and see if we could reason with her.' Still, it took quite a few people to hold her and she screamed and it was awful.

"But it was not until October, 1989, that she learned by accident, at the Orange County Children's Hospital parent support meeting, that the psychology department offered biofeedback.

At the time, 4½ year old Cory was the hospital's youngest biofeedback student.

But Burns was hopeful. Cory was eager to find a way to block the pain. Also the hospital's biofeedback programs—some displaying charts and colorful shapes, one depicting a small man climbing a mountain as the child's tension rose—seemed tailored toward kids, Burns said. And "Cory's pretty video-literate"—good at video games like Nintendo. "I thought this would be right up her alley."

And it was. After just two half-hour sessions with the biofeedback equipment, Cory had learned relaxation techniques, said Frank Carden, the hospital's director of health psychology. (Each session costs $65, and insurance companies typically pay for the treatment.)

In November when she had her next puncture, "she was a little stressed," her mother admitted. But instead of nurses holding her, Cory rested quietly on the procedure table.

"There was just one little scream. And it was over." Burns said.

How does Cory do biofeedback? Meeting with a reporter at her family's rustic home in Riverside's orange groves, the little girl—a typical 6 year old—made it clear that she would prefer to discuss her gray pony Moki, her Little Mermaid watch or her two toy ponies, Miss Sparkle and Miss Dawn, rather than biofeedback.

Still with her mother's prompting, Cory talked a little. Practicing biofeedback, she said, batting large brown eyes, "is just like you're trying to go to sleep."

By now, Cory has biofeedback down to a science, she and her mother said. About a week before each spinal tap, Cory visits the Orange County hospital for a half-hour refresher class in front of the video monitor.

And on the day of the needle stick, Burns stays by Cory's side, holding her hand, and coaching her on biofeedback techniques.

While Cory waits for the puncture, she and Burns also discuss an elaborate fantasy that they narrate together. In this waking dream, a stallion named Black Beauty gallops through the forest, carrying young Cory to a safe place—beyond pain.

"I just remember when I'm getting my pokes, I think about riding Black Beauty through the woods. And it's cool in the woods. And we go through the trees," Cory said.

Added Burns, "And when the poke is going to come, we think about a jump. And when it hurts a little, I say, "Breathe!" And it works.

Both Cory and Burns say they are delighted to have found biofeedback. Cory has even used it occasionally outside the hospital. Once, on the roller coaster at Castle Park in Riverside, they were both scared, Burns said, but Cory stayed calm, working her way through her terror by breathing deeply, relaxing her shoulders, practicing biofeedback.

Overall, Burns said, her only concern about biofeedback was that Cory didn't learn about this sooner.

"I don't know why this is such a well-kept secret," Burns said.

Whether it would work for children much younger than Cory, Burns said she didn't know. "But it's worth trying for Pete's sakes. These little guys—they don't know what's happening to them and biofeedback could give them something to do, give them some control over their pain," Burns said.[1]

There are numerous books and articles on biofeedback, chronic pain, stress-related symptoms, and self-help techniques. There are also home practice biofeedback devices, guided relaxation tapes, healing music tapes, and tapes that focus on the sounds of nature. Some tapes provide subliminal messages and some address a particular health problem. There are also videotapes that provide relaxing images and lecture programs. I believe that most of these self-help products are potentially very helpful, but I do not believe that healing is a "do it yourself project."

Each of us is directly and indirectly sustained by those relationships that facilitate healing. When our connections with touching, caring, loving, remembering, and other basic elements of living are diminished, it is difficult to maintain a healthy state. Books, tapes, and other resources provide valuable self-help resources, but they cannot make up for the void that is created when a healing partnership is missing.

Norman Cousins, in an article titled "First Word," addresses the issue of creating a partnership of healing. He points out how important it is for physicians and therapists to help each patient to develop his/her own resources for healing.

Today's physician may be steered away from methods that effectively prevent and treat disease, but the American people somewhere along the way have been misinformed on how to care for and interpret their own bodies. We have separated ourselves from essential knowledge about the workings of the human body, unaware of the resources waiting to be put to use.

We are not altogether helpless when facing serious illness, yet individuals are timid, uncertain, and insecure about the way their own bodies work. Increasingly, we become oblivious to the relationship between causes and effects, both in illness and in food health. We often equate pain with disease, instead of seeing it as the body's early warning system, calling attention to potential problems. Instead of learning how to interpret the signals, people grab the nearest painkiller. The warning signs are then ignored and the symptoms are treated, some allowing the problem to escalate. People need to be taught that the healing system is connected to the belief system—a belief in our own abilities to understand and help heal our bodies.

Confidence, determination, and a strong will to live are not a substitute for competent medical attention, but they do help create an environment in which medical service can aid the patient most effectively. It is not necessary to believe that every illness is reversible, it is necessary to reach out for the best—the best that the physician has to offer and the best within oneself. The predictions of experts about the course of illness have been proved wrong often enough to justify putting hope—the life force—to work. Feelings of remorse or guilt, if the effort should fail, are not as tragic as the feeling that not all resources were fully tapped.

With increased individual knowledge of the inner resources that can be mobilized in combating illness, with deeper understanding of the separate but interrelated roles of patient and physician, and with wider public acceptance of the need to participate more fully in public health policy, the stage can be set for reform where reform is called for and for bringing health costs within reasonable limits. The main objective, of course, is not to see how cheaply health care can be obtained but to ensure optimal health care throughout the entire society. A sensible and effective national health program, dedicated to the public health, can be both economical and productive.[2]

Notes

1. Lanie Jones, "Easing pain with mind over matter," *Los Angeles Times* (October 28, 1990), E1–E10.
2. Norman Cousins, "First Word," *Omni Magazine* (December, 1989), p. 6.

CHAPTER 20

The Healing Partnership and the Common World

Chronic pain and chronic symptoms originate from many sources, and it is often impossible to unravel the intricately entwined causal factors. I very much agree with Ivan Illich's perspective that a medical nemesis has been created by focusing on medical technology as an answer to suffering. He states:

> Within the last decade medical professional practice has become a major threat to health. Depression, infection, disability, dysfunction, and other specific iatrogenic diseases now cause more suffering than all accidents from traffic or industry. Beyond this, medical practice sponsors sickness by reinforcement of a morbid society which not only industrially preserves its defectives but breeds the therapist's client in cybernetic ways. Finally, the so-called health-professions have an indirect sickening power—a structurally health-denying effect. I want to focus on this last syndrome, which I designate as medical Nemesis. By transforming pain, illness, and death from a personal challenge into a technical problem, medical practice expropriates the potential of people to deal with their human condition in an autonomous way and becomes the source of a new kind of un-health.[1]

The issues that Ivan Illich poses are, I believe, even more timely than they were when he first presented them. There is more emphasis on self-regulation and psychoneuroimmunology, but I would venture to say that a majority of the population feels shut out of the opportunity to take advantage of modern medical technology and has very limited knowledge about how to care for their own health. They dwell in a vast health-care wasteland that affects the whole of society. It is not medical technology that teaches us about health and healing. We learn how to care for ourselves from those who care for us, and in some cases this may mean that we learn very little. As Illich states:

> Mankind evolved only because each of its individuals came into existence protected by various visible and individual cocoons. Each one knew the womb from which he had come, and oriented himself by the stars under which he was born. To be human and to become human, the individual of our species has to find his destiny in his own unique struggle with Nature and neighbour. He is on his own in the struggle, but the weapons and the rules and the style are given to him by the culture in which he grew up. Each culture is the sum of rules with which the individual could come to terms with pain, sickness and death—could interpret them and practice compassion amongst others faced by the same threats. Each culture set the myth, the rituals, the taboos, and the ethical standards needed to deal with the fragility of life—to explain the reason for pain, the dignity of the sick, and the role of dying or death.
>
> Cosmopolitan medical civilization denies the need for man's acceptance of these evils. Medical civilization is planned and organized to kill pain, to eliminate sickness, and to struggle against death . . .
>
> Man's consciously lived fragility, individuality, and relatedness make the experience of pain, of sickness, and of death an integral part of his life. The ability to live with this trio in autonomy is fundamental to his health . . . The level of public health corresponds to the degree to which the means and responsibility for coping with illness are distributed amongst the total population. This ability to cope can be enhanced but never replaced by medical intervention in the lives of people or the hygienic characteristics of the environment. That society which can reduce professional intervention to the minimum will provide the best conditions for health. The greater the potential for autonomous adaptation of self

and to others and to the environment, the less management of adaptation will be needed or tolerated.[2]

We learn from each other what it means to be human and this is best accomplished, in the words of Martin Buber, by "touching each other and comprehending all others and thus making mankind a true humanity." While I was in India, a man who spoke little English asked me if I was in pain. He could see that I did not feel well and that I was holding my stomach. After I told him that I did indeed have pain, he pointed to his chest and uttered the word "pain." We sat there silently, but at that moment we shared our common humanity. The cultural differences and the language barrier were still there, but for a time we were not just "other" but part of a shared humanity: This shows that all people have some common ground. I think that we are, at all times, a reflection from our own prism of being. We cannot escape the fact that we are the other, and yet we are also more than this. I know myself and I know the other only by that in me which meets the other. In "meeting" the other I sometimes share my own pain, and in doing so I share both my vulnerability and my strengths. I try not to burden the patient, but rather to impart the fact that life is a shared experience and that while we will remain separate beings we can touch and help each other from where we are. This is what technology cannot accomplish, and it is how we help each other to learn the "adaptation" skills that are necessary to cope with illness, pain, and the fragility of life.

Martin Buber states, "Every real happening of the spirit is meeting (*Begegnung*)." He asserts that we cannot grasp psychologically the relationship to the beloved person or any experience of the Thou. We must, he states, be ready to give up our method.[2] "The therapist deals with the patient as an individual, yet the sickness is a sickness of the between."

> The sicknesses of the soul are sicknesses of relationship. They can only be treated completely if I transcend the realm of the patient and add to it the world as well. If the doctor possessed super-human power, he would have to try to heal the relationship itself, to heal the "between . . . "[3]

When one is in pain, there is a need to heal the spirit. We usually think of healing as something that occurs between the helper and the one in need of help, but healing often occurs in the most unexpected ways. In her book *The Diary of a Pigeon Watcher*, Doris Schwerin chronicles her recovery from breast-cancer surgery. Her story is intertwined with the daily life of a pigeon family that lives on a ledge outside her apartment window. As she observes the daily life of this pigeon family, Doris Schwerin begins to confront her pain, fear, and sense of loss, and she also begins the process of healing.

> Before the cancer, Time was what I chose to waste. After the cancer, it nagged at me constantly, that to be profligate with Time was the ultimate degeneracy. Only a fool would not change under the circumstances . . . Then something most unexpected happened. I took refuge in someone else's Time, so as not to watch my own, dumbly. It was the middle of my five-year wait (the magic five years they give cancer patients to see whether they'll make it or not) that I shifted my attention from my own mortality to the more mysterious one of another of God's creatures. Of all things, pigeons! Dirty, ubiquitous, lowly pigeons. The meeting, greeting, flying, love making, mating, birthing, tending, talking, resting, sleeping, cooing; the storms, the wars, the victories and defeats, the devotions, the laughter—the fight for life and joy of flight— pushed me back into the center of myself. I rode their waves in slow recognition and was reminded of many forgotten things in this cold, stone city.[4]

Doris Schwerin's book is about healing. It shows how the layers build up over the years and reveals the necessity of healing both present and past wounds. I have found that Schwerin's book, as well as the writings of Oliver Sacks, Alice Walker, Maya Angelou, Elie Wiesel, Franz Kafka, and many, many others have spoken to me in ways that have helped me to confront my own need for healing. Those who share their life experiences share their common humanity. There is a healing power in the human spirit that is often released when one shares one's personal uniqueness.

My own strength, especially during times of sorrow or pain,

comes from what I have learned from those who have shared their life experiences with me. This is especially true with regard to my childhood. There were no "how to" lectures or presentations of a "blueprint of life" to guide me on my way. There were stories of death, life, joy, adversity, failure, success, anger, forgiveness, and love. This is a gift that we can share with one another, especially from generation to generation. Here we become the "I," but we are also brought into the "We."

When a therapist needs the patient, it is unlikely that healing will occur. But when the patient no longer needs the therapist it is likely that healing has occurred. The wounded have a double task. They need to participate in the healing of their woundedness, and they need to become free from their dependence on the healer. Buber states:

> The healer fashions in the fellow-soul a ground and a center in order that the soul that calls to him, as through a glass, into Being. The more fully and genuinely this ground and center is fashioned, the less does the appealing soul remain dependent upon the helper. But the less, too, does he fall back into psychologism.[5]

Doris Schwerin beautifully describes the healing that emerged as she was able to let go of her woundedness and to make peace with her parents and feel a sense of wholeness.

> I felt alive through the use of Time, and a woman who had come from their nest; that I no longer needed the ritual mask; and I had embraced its essence and would pass it on; and that I would never stop searching for a sense of Order within and beyond the circumference of our wounds, theirs and mine. Standing there in the bright Indian summer sun, I laughed out loud.[6]

Maya Angelou states, "Love affords wonder. And it is only love that gives one the liberty to go inside and see who am I really."[7]

Elaine Scarry, as we saw in Chapter 17, introduces the concept of restoring and/or creating a world. Pain and imagination are seen as providing a framing identity of man-as-creator. Work becomes the link to the world.

It is through this movement out into the world that the extreme privacy of the occurrence (both pain and imagining are invisible to anyone outside the boundaries of the person's body) begins to be sharable [sic], that sentience becomes social and thus acquires its distinctly human form.[8]

Martin Buber adds a needed dimension to Scarry's concept of restoring and/or creating a world. It is not primarily work, but the spoken word—the *logos*—that builds a common world.

Man has always had his experiences as I, his experiences with others, and with himself; but—it is as We, ever again as We, that he has constructed and developed a world out of his experiences. . . . Thus . . . in the midst of precipitous being, the human cosmos is preserved, guarded by its moulder, the human speech-with-meaning, the common logos. Thus the cosmos is preserved amid the changes of the world images. Man has always thought his thoughts as I, and as I he has transplanted his ideas into the firmament of the spirit, but as We he has ever raised them into being itself, in just that mode of existence that I call 'the between' or 'betweenness.' . . . We ourselves . . . as the ready and obedient bearers of the word, the logos, accord to the cosmos its reality which consists in being our world. Through us it becomes the shaped world of man, and only now does it deserve the name of cosmos as a total order, formed and revealed. Only through our service to the logos does the world become 'the same cosmos for all.' Thus and only thus do the waking, just in so far as they are awake, have in truth a single common world whose unity and community they work on in all real waking existence. . . . However, this working together is in no way to be conceived of as a team hitched to the great wagon: It is a strenuous tug of war for a wager, it is battle and strife. But in so far as it lets itself be determined by the logos it is a common battle and produces the common: out of the extremest tension, when it takes place in the service of the logos, arises ever anew the harmony of the lyre.[9]

The healing partnership helps to bring the individual back into the world as an "I." This is the first step toward recreating one's world, but it is not the completed task. The movement of going out into the world is a necessary step in moving from being an "I" to the creation of the "We." Martin Buber addresses this issue in his essay "What is Common to All."

> The genuine We is to be recognized in its objective existence, through the fact that in whatever of its parts it is regarded, an essential relation between person and person, between I and Thou, is always evident as actually or potentially existing. For the word always arises between an I and a Thou, and the element from which the We receives its life is speech, the communal speaking that begins in the midst of speaking to one another.[10]

To establish a sense of self, we must have our own ground from which to meet the other. This ground of being is established in the healing partnership. This is not the domain of the professional/patient relationship, but occurs whenever there is genuine dialogue between one person and another. In establishing our own ground of being there may be periods of turning inward, but if this inward quest becomes the goal, it will serve to create a distance between one's self and the world. If we are to partake in the building of a world, there must also be a movement into the world. This is not a passive joining of self and world, but a meeting that is built up in genuine communication. It is, to paraphrase Buber's words, a willingness to answer for the genuineness of our existence.

I once had a patient who had suffered a total loss of hearing when he was 8 years old. He was now 30 years old and suffering from multiple symptoms of stress. His main source of stress, he felt, was his workplace. He relied on lip-reading at work and his fellow employees and, in particular, his supervisor, often spoke to him in ways that made it very difficult for him to decipher what was being said. At times he was confused about some aspect of his work responsibilities, and at all times he felt excluded from the world of the other employees.

We worked together with the help of a sign interpreter and our communication flowed back and forth at a steady pace, but I was unable to be of help to this patient. He stated, "You will never understand my problem." I suggested seeking more support and help from the hearing-impaired community, but he quickly rejected this suggestion.

> You do not understand my problem. I was once a part of the hearing world, and that sets me apart from most of those who have been hearing-impaired from birth or early childhood. They can't understand my problems either. I don't fit into either world, and there isn't anything you can do for me.

For this patient there was no sense of having a ground of being. He felt completely shut out of the world and he could find no way to express in dialogue the pain and suffering that he was experiencing. His anger and frustration had spilled over into every aspect of his life and had driven him to retreat further into his own place of woundedness. His were wounds that he believed had been inflicted by the very world that I represented, and he did not see himself as belonging to that world.

Buber's interpretation of "What Is Common to All" is based on the teachings of Heraclitus. Heraclitus states: "Do not listen to me but to the *logos*." Buber adds his own commentary to this and other teachings of Heraclitus and states,

> Each soul does, of course, have its logos deep in itself, but the logos does not attain to its fullness in us but rather between us; for it means the eternal chance for speech to become true between men. Therefore it is common to them.[11]

Healing arises from the between, but often it is not the patient, but the professional who establishes a distance that creates an illusion that a "common logos" does not exist. Healing goes beyond the removal of symptoms. It addresses the human spirit, and it is everyone's domain. It has as its foundation the building of the world and this is what we all have in common.

We exclude others by discounting their voice, not hearing their words, failing to respond to their needs, and restricting the concept of "We" to a select few. This causes an injury to the spirit of the other which causes the other to retreat into his or her own woundedness. Like my hearing-impaired patient, they are no longer able to hear the call to respond and the "I" becomes atrophied. For this person a common *logos* does not exist. There is a silence that diminishes the existence of all people in the world. Buber states:

> Speech in its ontological sense was at all times present wherever men regarded one another in the mutuality of I and Thou; wherever one showed the other something in the world in such a way that from then on he began really to perceive it; wherever one gave another a sign in such a way that he could recognize the designated situation as he had not been able to before; wherever one communicated to the other his own experience in such a way that it penetrated the other's circle of experience and supplemented it as from within, so that from now on his perceptions were set within a world as they had not been before. All this flowing ever again into a great stream of reciprocal sharing of knowledge—this came to be and thus is the living We, the genuine We, which, when it fulfills itself, embraces the dead who once took part in colloquy and now take part in it through what they have handed down to posterity.[12]

Every child wants to be called into being, but when this does not occur he/she, like my hearing-impaired patient, may spend a lifetime shut out of the world. In sharing an early childhood memory, Elizabeth Cotton shared the importance of being personally addressed by another.

> I named myself. The first day I went to school, the teacher was calling roll and everybody was called a name. My parents didn't name me. They all called me Sis, you know. So when the teacher got to me, she said, "Li'l Sis, don't you have a name? What is it?" And I just said, "Elizabeth." I don't know where I got that name. So she put it down and I started being called Elizabeth.

This event is what Maurice Friedman refers to as a touchstone of reality.[13] The teacher's question evoked a response that established Elizabeth Cotton's right to exist as an "I," and to begin to create her own ground of being. She became a professional folk singer at the age of 65 and went on to win a Grammy award when she was 92 years old. I had the privilege of hearing Elizabeth Cotton perform at a small local concert. In sharing her music she shared her most important touchstone of reality. She also shared aspects of her life history and by doing so brought us into her world. This is speech in the ontological sense. My circle of experience was penetrated and my own world enhanced. Here spirit meets spirit and the "I" is lifted into the "We." This is how we build a world and begin to realize the possibility of a common cosmos.

When Two Sing

"When one person is singing and cannot lift his voice," said a Hasidic rabbi, "and another comes and sings with him, another who can lift his voice, then the first will be able to lift his voice. That," said the rabbi, "is the secret of the bond between spirit and spirit."[14]

In an article titled "The Littlest Victim," 5-year-old Jennifer Royal describes how she was shot by a man in her neighborhood, and how this same man also shot and killed her 8-year-old friend. She was one of the youngest witnesses to testify in an American courtroom, and she helped to convict the person who had both wounded her and killed her best friend.

During the interview, Jennifer poignantly describes her life in a world that is filled with crime, drugs, and violence. But she also shares her dreams of building another world, and her fears.

I'm going to school soon. That's what I want most. We are going to learn everything at school. . . . When I grow up I want to be one of those people in an office. A secretary. I will write letters to everyone who likes me. And I want to go to New York City and ride around on the bus with grandma and go in a big white limousine with a TV and radio and cookies and wine. . . . One time I dreamed, coming home from school, I saw a fox. I see him across the street. Everybody at home is asleep. He ate my arm up. He killed me with his mouth. I just shook my head. I said, "No! I don't want you to eat me up."[15]

To penetrate the circle of one's experience there must be dialogue. If this child's voice does not continue to be heard, she may suffer from a wounded spirit, and this type of pain is not easily healed. To build a common cosmos the circle of being must continually be expanded through dialogue. A closed world does not restore and/or create a world. It causes an atrophied center of being that destroys the self from within. The healing partnership opens up the possibility of "meeting" and of healing. This in turn opens up the possibility of restoring and/or creating a common world.

If the psychotherapist is satisfied to "analyse" the patient, i.e., to bring to light unknown factors from his microcosm, and set to some conscious work in life the energies which have been transformed by such an emergence then he/she may be successful in some repair work. At best, he or she may help a soul that is diffused and poor in structure to collect and order itself to some extent. But the real matter, the regeneration of an atrophied personal center, will not be achieved. This can only be done by one who grasps the buried latent unity of the suffering soul with the great glance of the doctor: and this can only be attained in the person-to-person attitude of a partner, not by the consideration and examination of an object.[16]

Notes

1. Ivan Illich, "Medical Nemesis."
2. Ibid., pp. 28–32.
3. Martin Buber, *A Believing Humanism: My Testament 1902–1965*. Translated by Maurice Friedman (New Jersey: Humanities Press, 1967), p. 150.
4. Doris Schwerin, *The Diary of a Pigeon Watcher* (New York: Paragon House Publishers, 1987), p. 9.
5. Maurice Friedman, *Martin Buber's Life and Work 1878–1923* (New York, E. P. Dutton, 1981), p. 353.
6. Doris Schwerin, *The Diary of a Pigeon Watcher* (New York: Paragon House Publishers, 1987), p. 288.
7. Maya Angelou, *I Dream A World: Portraits of Black Women Who Changed America*, edited by Brian Lenker (New York: Stewart, Tabori and Chang, 1989), p. 162.
8. Elaine Scarry, *The Body in Pain* (New York: Oxford University Press, 1985), p. 170.

9. Martin Buber, *The Knowledge of Man* (New York: Harper and Row, 1965), pp. 105–107.

10. Ibid., p. 106.

11. Ibid., p. 104.

12. Ibid., p. 106.

13. Elizabeth Cotton, *I Dream A World*, edited by Brian Lenker (New York: Stewart Tabori and Chang, 1989), p. 156.

14. Martin Buber, *Tales of the Hasidim: The Early Masters* (New York: Schocken Books, 1946), p. 133.

15. Valerie Gladstone, "The littlest victim," *Life Magazine* (Fall, 1990), pp. 16–18.

16. Martin Buber, *I and Thou*, translated by Ronald Gregor Smith (New York: Charles Scribner's Sons, 1958) pp. 132–133.

Index

297